SPORT AND EXERCISE MEDICINE OSCEs

SPORT AND EXERCISE MEDICINE OSCEs

An Essential Revision Guide

Natalie F. Shur
MBChB, BMedSci (Hons), MRes, MRCP (UK), MFSEM (UK)

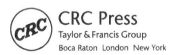

CRC Press
Taylor & Francis Group
Boca Raton London New York

CRC Press is an imprint of the
Taylor & Francis Group, an **informa** business

First edition published 2022
by CRC Press
6000 Broken Sound Parkway NW, Suite 300, Boca Raton, FL 33487-2742

and by CRC Press
2 Park Square, Milton Park, Abingdon, Oxon, OX14 4RN

© 2022 Taylor & Francis Group, LLC

CRC Press is an imprint of Taylor & Francis Group, LLC

Library of Congress Cataloging-in-Publication Data

Names: Shur, Natalie, author.
Title: Sport and exercise medicine OSCEs : an essential revision guide / Natalie Shur.
Description: First edition. | Boca Raton : CRC Press, 2022. | Includes bibliographical references and index. | Summary: "A study guide for those studying Sport and Exercise Medicine and sitting examinations. Divided into sections based on the main topics that arise in SEM OSCEs, the book provides both core knowledge and practical tips to ensure a successful performance by the examinee in every station. Written for those about to sit a postgraduate examination in sport and exercise medicine, or those enrolled on a postgraduate certificate or masters course in the specialty will value this book. Doctors, physiotherapists, sports therapists, podiatrists, nurses, and undergraduate students"— Provided by publisher.
Identifiers: LCCN 2021025799 (print) | LCCN 2021025800 (ebook) | ISBN 9780367706784 (paperback) | ISBN 9780367757243 (hardback) | ISBN 9781003163701 (ebook)
Subjects: MESH: Sports Medicine | Exercise Therapy | United Kingdom | Outline
Classification: LCC QP301 (print) | LCC QP301 (ebook) | NLM QT 18.2 | DDC 612/.044—dc23
LC record available at https://lccn.loc.gov/2021025799
LC ebook record available at https://lccn.loc.gov/2021025800

ISBN: 9780367757243 (hbk)
ISBN: 9780367706784 (pbk)
ISBN: 9781003163701 (ebk)

DOI: 10.1201/9781003163701

Typeset in Utopia
by KnowledgeWorks Global Ltd.

Contents

Foreword

A career in sport and exercise medicine has provided me with the privilege of working in a specialty in evolution. This evolution has involved specialty recognition, the creation of the Faculty of Sport and Exercise Medicine and with it the setting of standards. Such standards in medicine necessarily involve curriculum and assessment, thus examinations.

As the only text on the market for Sport and Exercise Medicine OSCEs, this excellent book will be an invaluable guide to those studying sport and exercise medicine and for those sitting examinations. Whilst specifically targeted at the OSCE, this book will have much wider appeal. Through its 18 clearly structured chapters not only does it provide a useful revision guide for the sport and exercise medicine curriculum, but also an invaluable guide to help one's thinking and behaviours on exams and in clinical situations.

The author is a highly impressive and accomplished academic trainee in Sport and Exercise Medicine. She is a working mother, clinician and researcher. She is extremely good in exam situations, being awarded the 2020 Macleod Medal as the candidate with the highest mark in both diets of the Membership examination, and is thus well-placed to author this book. I first met Natalie when she was considering a career in Sport and Exercise Medicine – she, with her colleagues, represent the future of this wonderful specialty of medicine.

Dr Mark E Batt
Consultant Sport and Exercise Medicine
Hon Prof School of Medicine
University of Nottingham

Preface

Education is a progressive discovery of our own ignorance.

Will Durrant

To teach is to learn twice.

Joseph Joubert

The inevitable Clinical Objective Structured Clinical Examination (OSCE) is a much anticipated and anxiety-provoking final obstacle in any clinician's path to the promised land on the other side. But in such a new and evolving specialty such as Sport and Exercise Medicine, OSCEs have always seemed even more mysterious and elusive somehow.

The idea for this book came about whilst revising for the Faculty of Sport and Exercise Medicine Part 2 Diploma Exam (twice; my original exam date was postponed due to the COVID-19 pandemic). Although there are several books that present a broad overview of Sport and Exercise Medicine, none specifically focus on how to pass an OSCE in the subject, what sorts of stations you might expect or how to approach revision in one text. Hence, in my frustration, I decided to write my own and try to present in a concise and pragmatic way some of the pearls and pitfalls I picked up along the way. This book contains everything you want and need to know for your exam in one accessible place.

The aim of this book is to provide the reader with the tools to confidently and competently pass an OSCE in Sport and Exercise Medicine. The book is divided into sections based on the main topics that arise in Sport and Exercise Medicine OSCEs, with essential core knowledge and practical tips to produce a fluid and confident performance in every station. It is directed at those about to sit a postgraduate examination in Sport and Exercise Medicine or those enrolled in a postgraduate certificate or master's course in Sport and Exercise Medicine. It will be of benefit to doctors and allied healthcare professionals, such as physiotherapists, sports therapists, podiatrists and nurses, as well as undergraduate students. This book will also be useful to the young clinician who is just starting and wants to build their confidence in musculoskeletal assessment and presenting to seniors.

All of the material in this book, coupled with intensive practice with peers and clinical experience was the foundation for me to be able to successfully pass the ever-elusive OSCE in Sport and Exercise Medicine. It is an exciting time to be practising Sport and Exercise Medicine, with the evidence base changing on a daily basis. The more I learn, the more I realise how much I don't know. However, I hope this text imparts just a sprinkle of wisdom to help you on your way in your journey.

Acknowledgements

Passing any OSCE exam and subsequently writing a book on how to pass it is not possible on your own and I am immensely grateful to my peers and colleagues for all their support and help. I would particularly like to thank my excellent colleagues Rob Barker-Davies and Romila Bahl, who were my revision partners and who were equally successful in passing the exam the first time. I would like to thank Philippa Turner, Pumi Seneratne and Jill Neale and all of the other consultants and trainees for their revision sessions, tips and advice.

I am grateful to Arieff Abuhassan for his expertise in putting together Chapter 18 and providing excellent images and timely support. I am grateful to all those at CRC Press/Taylor & Francis for helping to make my idea a reality and in taking on such a text in a relatively niche specialty. Thank you to Miranda Bromage and Samantha Cook for always answering my queries at any time of the day during the writing and publishing process.

I am forever grateful to my family, in particular my parents, for their eternal encouragement and support in everything I do. Special thanks go to my husband Nick, who has been with me through more exams and higher degrees than he cares to remember and who continues to be my rock. Any partner of a medic quite frankly deserves a medal. Finally, I am fortunate to have several inspirational women in my life who motivate me to push myself every day. This book is dedicated to two, in particular, Rose and Eva.

Natalie F. Shur

Abbreviations

ΔΔ	differential diagnosis
A&E	Accident and Emergency
ACEi	angiotensin converting enzyme inhibitor
ACJ	acromioclavicular joint
ACL	anterior cruciate ligament
ACSM	American College of Sport and Exercise Medicine
ADAMS	Anti-Doping Administration and Management System
ADL	activities of daily living
AEDs	automated external defibrillators
AIIS	anterior inferior iliac spine
AIN	anterior interosseous nerve
AIOS	acquired instability overuse syndrome
ALP	alkaline phosphatase
ALSG	Advanced Life Support Group
AMBRI	Atraumatic, Multidirectional, Bilateral, Rehabilitation, Inferior capsular shift
AMS	acute mountain sickness
AMSSM	American Medical Society for Sports Medicine
ANA	antinuclear antibody
APB	abductor pollicis brevis
APL	abductor pollicis longus
ARDS	acute respiratory distress syndrome
ASIA	American Spinal Cord Injury Association
ASIS	anterior superior iliac spine
ATFL	anterior talofibular ligament
ATFL	anterior tibiofibular ligament
ATMMiF	Advanced Trauma Medical Management in Football
AVN	avascular necrosis
BASDAI	Bath Ankylosing Spondylitis Disease Activity Index
BESS	British Elbow and Shoulder Society
BJHS	benign joint hypermobility syndrome
BMBS	Bachelor of Medicine and Bachelor of Surgery
BMD	bone mineral density
BMI	body mass index
BP	blood pressure
BSI	bone stress injury
CAP	chest, abdomen, pelvis
CAQ	Certificate of Added Qualification
CASEM	Canadian Academy of Sport and Exercise Medicine
CBT	cognitive behavioural therapy
CC	coracoclavicular

CECS	chronic exertional compartment syndrome
CEO	common extensor origin
CFL	calcaneofibular ligament
CFO	common flexor origin
CHD	oronary heart disease
CK	creatine kinase
CMC	carpometacarpal
CMO	Chief Medical Officer
CMV	cytomegalovirus
CPR	cardiopulmonary resuscitation
CRP	C-reactive protein
CSF	cerebrospinal fluid
CT	computed tomography
CTC	Certificate of Completion of Training
CTE	chronic traumatic encephalopathy
CTS	carpal tunnel syndrome
CV	cardiovascular
CXR	chest X-ray
DCI	decompression illness
DDH	developmental dysplasia of the hip
DEXA	dual energy X-ray absorptiometry
DHEAs	dehydroepiandrosterone sulphate
DIC	disseminated intravascular coagulation
DIP	distal interphalangeal joint
DKA	diabetic ketoacidosis
DM	diabetes mellitus
DMARD	disease modifying anti-rheumatic drug
DVLA	Driver and Vehicle Licensing Agency
DVT	deep vein thrombosis
EBV	Epstein-Barr virus
ECG	electrocardiogram
ECRB	extensor carpi radialis brevis
ECSW	extra corporeal shock wave
ECU	extensor carpi ulnaris
ED	eating disorders
ED	extensor digitorum
EDL	extensory digitorum longus
EDS	Ehlers-Danlos syndrome
EHL	extensor hallucis longus
EI	extensor indicis
EIB	exercise-induced bronchoconstriction
EILO	exercise-induced laryngeal obstruction
EMG	electromyography
ENT	ear, nose and throat
EPB	extensor pollicis brevis
EPL	extensor pollicis longus
ER	external rotation

ESR	erythrocyte sedimentation rate	**LH**	luteinising hormone
ESWT	extra-corporal shock wave therapy	**LMN**	lower motor neuron
EVH	eucapnic voluntary hyperpnoea	**LOC**	loss of consciousness
FABER	flexion abduction and external rotation	**LRTI**	lower respiratory tract infection
		MC	metacarpal
FADIR	flexion adduction and internal rotation	**MCL**	medial collateral ligament
		MCP	metacarpophalangeal joints
FAI	femoroacetabular impingement	**MDT**	multidisciplinary team
FBC	full blood count	**MFSEM**	Membership of the Faculty of Sport and Exercise Medicine, UK
FCR	flexor carpi radialis		
FCU	flexor carpi ulnaris	**MI**	myocardial infarction
FDP	flexor digitorum profundus	**MILS**	manual in-line stabilisation
FDS	flexor digitorum superficialis	**MIMMS**	Major Incident Medical Management and Support
FeNO	fractional exhaled nitric oxide		
FEV	forced expiratory volume	**MoCA**	Montreal Cognitive Assessment
FH	family history	**MOI**	mechanism of injury
FHL	flexor hallucis longus	**MPFL**	medial patellofemoral ligament
FPL	flexor pollicis longus	**MRC**	Medical Research Council
FSEM	Faculty of Sport and Exercise Medicine	**MRI**	magnetic resonance imaging
		MS	multiple sclerosis
FSH	follicle-stimulating hormone	**MSK**	musculoskeletal
FVC	forced vital capacity	**MT**	metatarsal
GCS	Glasgow Coma Scale	**MTJ**	musculotendinous junction
GDPR	General Data Protection Regulation	**MTP**	metatarsophalangeal
GIRD	glenohumeral internal rotation deficit	**MTSS**	medial tibial stress syndrome
GMC	Good Medical Council	**MVP**	mitral valve prolapse
GnRH	gonadotropin-releasing hormone	**NAC**	N-acetylcysteine
GORD	gastroesophageal reflux disease	**NaTHNaC**	National Travel Health Network and Centre
GP	General Practitioner		
GTN	glyceryl trinitrate	**NCS**	nerve conduction studies
GUM	genitourinary medicine	**NEXUS**	National Emergency X-Radiography Utilization Study
HACE	high altitude cerebral oedema		
HAPE	high altitude pulmonary oedema	**NICE**	National Institute for Health and Care Excellence
HBA1c	haemoglobin A1c		
HCM	hypertrophic cardiomyopathy	**NM**	neuromuscular
HDL	high density lipoprotein	**NOF**	neck of femur
HIA	Head Injury Assessment	**NP**	nasopharyngeal
HIV	human immunodeficiency virus	**NSAIDs**	non-steroidal anti-inflammatory drugs
IBD	inflammatory bowel disease		
IBD	inflammatory bowel disease	**NWB**	non–weight-bearing
IC	Intracranial	**OA**	osteoarthritis
ICE	ideas, concerns and expectations	**OGTT**	oral glucose tolerance test
ICP	intra-compartmental pressure	**OP**	opponens pollicis
ICS	inhaled corticosteroids	**OP**	oropharyngeal
IMMFP	Immediate Medical Management of the Field of Play	**ORIF**	open reduction internal fixation
		OSA	obstructive sleep apnoea
IPAQ	International Physical Activity Questionnaire	**OSCE**	Objective Structured Clinical Examination
ITB	iliotibial band	**OT**	occupational therapy
JIA	juvenile idiopathic arthritis	**OTC**	over the counter
LABA	long-acting β2 agonist	**PALS**	Patient Advice and Liaison Service
LAME	lateral aspect of the medical epicondyle	**PAR-Q+**	Physical Activity Readiness Questionnaire
LBP	lower back pain	**PCL**	posterior cruciate ligament
LCL	lateral collateral ligament	**PCOS**	polycystic ovarian syndrome
LDH	lactate dehydrogenase	**PDFS**	proton density fat saturated
LDL	low density lipoprotein	**PEF**	peak expiratory flow
LFT	liver function test	**PEFR**	peak expiratory flow rate

PET	positron emission tomography	SOCRATES	Site, Onset, Character, Radiation, Associated symptoms, Time/duration, Exacerbating/relieving factors, Severity
PFA	Professional Football Association		
PFJ	patellofemoral joint		
PFP	patellofemoral pain		
PHICIS	Pre-Hospital Immediate Care in Sport	SOL	space-occupying lesion
PIN	posterior interosseous nerve	SOPs	standard operating procedures
PIP	proximal interphalangeal joint	SpA	spondyloarthropathy
PLC	posterolateral corner	SPECT	single-photon emission computerized tomography
PMH	past medical history		
PNX	pneumothorax	SSRI	serotonin reuptake inhibitor
POLICE	protect, optimal loading, ice, compression, elevation	STI	sexually transmitted infection
		STIR	short-tau inversion recovery
PPE	pre-participation evaluation	SUFE	superior upper femoral epiphysis
PR	per rectum	T1WI	T1-weighted imaging
PREPARE	Provision, Equipment, Personnel, Administration, Read	T2DM	type II diabetes mellitus
		T2WI	T2-weighted imaging
PT	patellar tendinopathy	TB	tuberculosis
PTFL	posterior talofibular ligament	TED	thrombo-embolus deterrent
PVD	peripheral vascular disease	TEPID-OIL	Training, Equipment, Personnel, Information, Doctrine and concepts, Organisation, Infrastructure and Logistics
PXE	pseudoxanthoma elasticum		
RC	rotator cuff		
RCT	randomised controlled trial		
RED-S	relative energy deficiency in sport	TFCC	triangular fibrocartilage complex
RF	radio frequency	TFT	thyroid function test
ROM	range of movement	TOS	thoracic outlet syndrome
RPE	rate of perceived exertion	TT-TG	tibial tubercle to trochlear groove
RTP	return to play	TUBS	Traumatic, Unilateral, Bankart lesion, Surgery
S&C	strength and conditioning		
SABA	short-acting β_2 agonist	TUE	therapeutic use exemption
SCD	sudden cardiac death	UCL	ulnar collateral ligament
SCI	spinal cord injury	UKAD	UK Anti-Doping
SCJ	sternoclavicular joint	URTI	upper respiratory tract infection
SEM	sport and exercise medicine	US	ultrasound
SIADH	syndrome of inappropriate secretion of antidiuretic hormone	UTI	urinary tract infection
		VAS	visual analogue scale
SIJ	sacroiliac joint	VF	ventricular fibrillation
SLAP	superior labrum anterior to posterior	VIBE	volumetric interpolated breath-hold examination
SLE	systemic lupus erythematosus		
SLJ	Sinding-Larsen-Johansson	VL	vastus lateralis
SLR	straight leg raise	VT	ventricular tachycardia
SMHAT	Sport Mental Health Assessment Tool	WADA	World Anti-Doping Agency
SOB	shortness of breath	WCC	white cell count

1 How to prepare for an OSCE examination in SEM

INTRODUCTION

If you have passed the first written part of the exam, you have demonstrated that you have the breadth of knowledge required to practice sport and exercise medicine (SEM) in theory. The aim of the objective structured clinical examination (OSCE) is the clinical application of this knowledge and the assessment of several parts of the curriculum that cannot be demonstrated in a written exam. This includes not only your knowledge of SEM but also your communication skills, clinical decision making, investigation interpretation and pitch-side safety as well as professionalism and behaviour. You won't fail for not knowing minutiae. The exam is ultimately assessing your ability to practice SEM safely and competently, being able to think widely in constructing a differential diagnosis and management plan, and in being able to communicate with patients accurately and professionally. Find out the format of the particular exam you will be sitting including the length of the stations and base your practice around that.

This book has been put together to aid you in your revision. It will cover the main topics that arise in SEM OSCEs and provides key knowledge and practical information to perform well on the day. For ease, this book has been divided into three parts covering the main types of stations that may arise: Part A covering history and examination and clinical cases (Chapters 2–10), Part B covering communication stations (Chapters 11–15) and Part C covering emergencies (Chapters 16 and 17). Finally, there is a radiology chapter summarising the radiological features of key diagnoses in the specialty. Several topics have been written as though they are an OSCE station with a 'clinical vignette' at the beginning similar to the ones you may receive before each station in your actual exam.

HOW TO APPROACH OSCE REVISION

The first step is to carefully research the format of the specific exam you are sitting, including the length of stations, topics covered and skills being assessed so that you can focus your revision. Practice in groups as much as possible, ideally with candidates with the same level of knowledge or better than your own. Groups of three or four people are best, with one person being the candidate, one person being the 'patient' and the other the examiner. Critique each other constructively at the end of each practice station. Communication-type stations can be practiced online in groups if necessary, but examination and emergency stations are best practiced face to face. Practice timed stations so you start to automatically get a feel for how long the stations will be. If the station is a 10-minute examination station, aim to complete the exam in approximately 7–8 minutes. Don't waste the first 3 minutes nervously chattering away as this will not pick up points. You will need at least 2–3 months whilst working clinically to prepare for an OSCE. Get registrars and consultants to critique your examination technique and grill you. The key is to practice scenarios *ad nauseum*.

In the United Kingdom, The Membership in SEM exam is designed to assess the knowledge, skills, competence and professional attitudes required of a doctor who wishes to practice as a SEM physician in the United Kingdom. Candidates must have passed the Faculty of Sport and Exercise Medicine (FSEM) Membership Part 1 written exam before being eligible to apply for Part 2. The exam can be sat by doctors with a medical qualification acceptable to the UK General Medical Council for Full or Provisional Registration or to the Medical Council in Ireland for Full or Temporary Registration and either:

- Be a current trainee in SEM.
- Have a minimum of 2 years clinical practice or postgraduate training after obtaining full registration and must have competence in cardiopulmonary resuscitation and pre-hospital care.

Successfully completing Parts 1 and 2 of the exam provides formal accreditation in the field of SEM. The Membership exam is essential for candidates wishing to:

- Obtain a Certificate of Completion of Training (CTC) in SEM.

DOI: 10.1201/9781003163701-1

- Apply for membership of the Faculty of Sport and Exercise Medicine, UK (MFSEM). It is also part of the requirements for a Fellowship application.

The FSEM Part 2 exam is run annually and consists of 12×10-minute stations, approximately a third of which are core skills (emergency scenarios), a third are clinical skills (musculoskeletal) and a third of which are oral examination stations (communication and ethics). Practice all three during your preparation. One station may be a preparatory station prior to a communication station (e.g. team travel planning scenario).

The Australasian College of Sport and Exercise Medicine Part II exam is a clinical exam typically sat in the final year of higher specialist training for sport and exercise medicine registrars. Candidates must pass the Part I exam to sit the Part II exam. The clinical exam is approximately 4 hours in duration and includes the following three Assessment Stations with rest periods in between (in any order):

1. Long case examination – 30-minute history and examination time with patient, 10-minute preparation (patient not in room) followed by a 20-minute assessment time with examiners (patient not in room) to present the case to the examiners, discuss investigations and management and answer relevant questions on the case.
2. Short case examinations – 45-minute session where a number of different cases/patients are examined.
3. Viva examination – 30-minute session covering various areas to assess clinical and medical knowledge, investigations, equipment and management.

The Canadian Academy of Sport and Exercise Medicine (CASEM) clinical exam comprises 18–20 OSCE stations. At each station, the candidate is asked to carry out a specific task or series of tasks, e.g. take a history and examine a patient with a specific problem, council an athlete or carry out an examination appropriate to the clinical situation. Pre-set standards are used as the basis for an objective evaluation of performance. Candidates must have a minimum of 2 years of independent medical practice, or a Fellow of the Royal College of Physicians and Surgeons or College of Family Physicians of Canada and have completed a 1-year Sport Medicine fellowship recognised by a University Faculty of Medicine Program. The program must include documented participation of 50 hours of team/sport/event coverage.

The American Medical Society for Sports Medicine (AMSSM) has a Certificate of Added Qualifications (CAQ) written exam, and Fellowship programs use OSCEs as part of their assessment during a fellows' training. In order to apply, candidates need to maintain their Family Medicine Certification, complete of a minimum 12 months of full-time training in an accredited Sports Medicine Fellowship Program and pass the Sports Medicine Certification Examination.

Numerous universities internationally run MSc or postgraduate diploma courses in SEM and feature an OSCE exam as part of their assessment. In countries where SEM is not a registered medical specialty, often an MSc in SEM is recognised by the home council. Entry requirements vary by institution, but typical entry requirements include a 2:1 in a relevant degree like Physiotherapy, Sports Therapy and other allied health sciences, or a Pass on a Bachelor of Medicine and Bachelor of Surgery degree (BMBS, MBBS, or equivalent). Historically some institutions running SEM MSc's also include anatomy stations in the OSCE involving anatomical prosections. This book will not specifically cover anatomy, as this knowledge is predominantly assessed during written exams. The emphasis is on you to find out the exact format of the OSCE used at your institution.

If your training programme in SEM is evaluated using continual assessment, e.g. comprising of Case-Based Discussions, then hopefully this book should give you the foundations to confidently assess and present cases in a logical, fluid and considered fashion.

THE DAY OF THE EXAM

Arrange travel and accommodation in good time. Ask for study leave with 6 weeks' notice and arrange any swaps for on-calls if required. If you are taking the exam at a distant location, it may be worth arriving the day before to avoid any stressful on-the-day travel delays and make sure you know how to get to the venue. Get a good night's sleep the evening before, ideally child-free, and bring some water and a snack with you on the day. You may be required to act out resuscitation in an acute scenario so make sure you wear comfortable but smart clothing.

Make sure you *read the question*. If not an acute station, it is normally either a communication station in which the history is key, or a station with a brief history with examination and discussion of management plan. If the latter, do not spend half the time taking a detailed history. You will not earn points. Be open minded and flexible in your approach; if in the course of a shoulder examination, it becomes apparent that the cervical spine is the culprit, switch your 'shoulder' exam to upper limb neurological exam and rule out red flags.

STATIONS WITH MANAGEMENT PLANS

In some stations you will be required to discuss a rehabilitation management plan of an athlete with a particular injury or problem. It's normally good to structure your answer and divide your answer into several parts to guide the consultation. SEM is a specialty that heavily involves the Multidisciplinary Team (MDT) so include this and think holistically regarding management, rather than solely focussing on musculoskeletal (MSK) rehabilitation or interventions, e.g. dietician referral if obese. In addition, you will pick up points for knowing specific examples of exercises rather than generically saying you would refer to physiotherapy. For example, describing specific rotator cuff strengthening exercises after a Superior Labrum Anterior to Posterior (SLAP) tear. Below is an example of how to frame your management plans, but you may want to devise your own framework to use:

1. Acute stage
   a. Activity modification
   b. Analgesia
   c. Restore range of movement (ROM), and normal gait and reduce swelling – e.g. ROM exercises
   d. Education of the patient about injury
   e. Maintain cardiovascular (CV) fitness
   f. Address relevant risk factors: nutrition, biomechanical, podiatry, training load, surfaces
2. Conditioning phase
   a. Resisted exercises, progressively increase sets and reps
   b. Progress to functional movements and later on plyometric
   c. Return to running programme
   d. Dietician involvement – if stress fracture related to relative energy deficiency in sport (RED-S), for example
   e. Athlete to join all team training and meetings
   f. Sports psychology support if necessary
3. Return to play phase
   a. Full ROM and strength
   b. Attending non-contact training before full contact
   c. Psychologically ready

Finally, put a plan in place for preventative measures to reduce risk of re-injury, e.g. strength and conditioning (S&C) throughout season, training load monitoring or technique adaptation.

EXAMINERS' QUESTIONS

If you find yourself being asked niche questions on physiology or a particular academic paper, this is normally a good sign, and they are pushing you to see the extent of your knowledge. Don't panic. If you don't know the answer, say so, but don't make things up. The examiners aren't there to deliberately trip you up. Communicate with the examiners with conviction in your answers.

PART A

History and examination and clinical cases

2 History and examination

INTRODUCTION

Taking a history is the most important diagnostic tool in a physician's repertoire. They say that if you allow the patient to talk for long enough, they will tell you the diagnosis. Unfortunately, in an objective structured clinical examination (OSCE), and indeed in the timed pressured environment of modern clinical practice, you are rarely afforded such time. If you are given a clinical station where history and examination have equal weighting, make sure you leave enough time to demonstrate both skills. Start with open questioning then move to closed questions to rule out wider differentials. If the patient mentions something unusual, ask them to explain further as there may be a hidden agenda in addition to the bread-and-butter musculoskeletal diagnosis you may be presented with, e.g. psychological or social issues. By the time you come to lay a hand on the patient to examine them you should already have a list of differential diagnoses in your head and then you can spend the examination ruling in or ruling out your hypotheses. You should also ensure you consider red flags and address this in your assessment. The following recommended history and examinations are lengthier than you may be able to achieve in an OSCE station. The real skill lies in selecting the right questions and examination manoeuvres to perform depending on the scenario, which requires a flexibility of mind, and only comes with clinical experience and practice *ad nauseum* with peers.

GENERAL TIPS

General tips for history taking and communication

For history taking it is advantageous to adopt the 'open to closed' question approach. Let the patient explain in their own words with a general opener then drill down to specifics using closed questions.

Contextualise their symptoms with regards to their occupation and physical activity or sport. It is essential to take a training history and a nutritional and menstrual history (if female) to identify potential causes for an injury such as training load spikes or relative energy deficiency in sport. There might be a 'hidden agenda' so always explore the patients' ideas, concerns and expectations (ICE). Think widely in terms of differentials; is this young footballer with a swollen knee presenting for the first time with a seronegative arthropathy or a reactive arthritis? If so, a brief sexual history is called for. Building a rapport, fluency of consultation and professionalism will earn you points, as will keeping to time.

General tips for examination

The sequences of examination in this book are a suggestion only, and are adaptable to your individual methods. Each doctor you ask will have a slightly different sequence of examination. Find your own way and stick with it and practice it until it becomes automated. The main thing is to have a fluid and competent examination which elicits the necessary findings without omitting key features and without causing pain to the patient. At the start of each station, wash your hands and identify the patient. Ask permission to examine the patient at the beginning and thank them at the end. If you have to position the patient to perform a manoeuvre, then ask politely. Always ensure adequate exposure for the examination you are performing. Develop your opening patter so that it is automated and concise 'Hello, my name is Dr Smith. I have been asked to examine your knee today. Would that be OK? Do you have any pain before I begin?' You may not have time to examine the good and injured side, but at least say you would compare and state at the end you would examine the joint above and the joint below. Verbalise what the examiner cannot see you do. If you have a lot to get through in an examination, don't be surprised if examiner moves you through certain parts of the

DOI: 10.1201/9781003163701-3

examination which is not being assessed. The special tests have been listed where they are appropriate to perform but they have not been detailed. You should be comfortable and familiar with performing all of the special tests listed in this book and know what they are specifically testing.

Presenting your findings

Some stations may require you to present a differential diagnosis to the examiner. In other stations, you will have to explain to the patient your diagnosis and plan.

Presenting your findings to the examiner

This can be the hardest part of an OSCE. Try to summarise your findings in 2–3 sentences and don't waffle.

- Turn to the examiner to present your findings. If you are guilty of overusing your limbs to illustrate your findings, stand with your hands behind your back to stop you pointing to the area you might be describing nervously. Don't be tempted to look back to the patient to remind yourself.
- If you know the diagnosis, then state what the diagnosis is and justify this with a list of positive findings and important negative findings.
  - E.g. The findings on history and examination are consistent with a diagnosis of lumbar stress fracture of the pars interarticularis. This is supported by pain on lumbar extension with a positive stork test, pain to palpation over the L4 pars and paraspinal muscle tightness. Important negatives are a lack of rest pain and normal neurology.
- If you are unsure of the diagnosis, don't panic. List the positive findings and pertinent negatives and then state what your top diagnosis is, followed by a list of differentials.
  - E.g. This patient has flexion-related lumbar spine pain with morning stiffness. On examination there is a reduced range of lumbar flexion and lateral flexion and pain over the left sacroiliac joint (SIJ). Important negatives are no evidence of psoriasis or other joint disease. My top differential is possible seronegative lumbar spine disease such as ankylosing spondylitis, but I would also consider other causes of a sacroiliitis such as infection or trauma or mechanical back pain.
- A coherent initial presentation like the above naturally leads the examiner to ask about your initial investigations and management. Start with simple investigations first, e.g. urine dip, then move onto bloods, then imaging and then additional special tests. Stating

magnetic resonance imaging (MRI) as your first-line investigation does not show much clinical acumen.

- E.g. To investigate a potential tibial stress fracture in this patient, firstly I would like to perform some simple bloods tests including FBC, U&E, LFTs, bone profile and TFTs. I would consider anti-TTG antibodies to screen for coeliac screen if symptomatic. I would then move to imaging which, given it is an early presentation X-rays are likely to be negative so I would perform an MRI, for which I would be looking for bone marrow oedema on T2-weighted imaging (T2WI)

Explaining your findings to the patient

Don't use medical jargon. Always ask if they have any questions and in management plans try to safety net yourself by organising follow-up plans for review. Involve the multidisciplinary team (MDT) if appropriate and explore the patient's concerns. Familiarise yourself with seminal papers or consensus statements which guide current best management for certain conditions, e.g. anterior cruciate ligament (ACL) management or concussion.

SHOULDER

"Ellie is a 21-year-old national swimmer with a 2-year history of bilateral shoulder pain. She trains 5 days per week, freestyle stroke and has a big meet at the end of the year. Her pain is non-responsive to simple analgesia. She has no history of trauma. Please examine this patient."

History

History of presenting complaint

- Onset of symptoms – acute onset or a chronic/insidious onset
- Pain (Use SOCRATES; Site, Onset, Character, Radiation, Associated symptoms, Time/duration, Exacerbating/Relieving factors, Severity)
- Site of pain is important in the shoulder
  - Acromioclavicular joint (ACJ)
  - Bicipital groove
  - Vague – rotator cuff (RC)
  - Deltoid – supraspinatus
  - Diffuse – osteoarthritis (OA) or adhesive capsulitis
- Any features of instability? Ask if they are hypermobile or 'double jointed'
- Mechanical symptoms such as clicking or clunking?
- What mechanism/position shoulder was in at time of injury?

- Exacerbating activity or position
- Pain at night – think rotator cuff or adhesive capsulitis
- Neurological symptoms such as paraesthesia or weakness
- Any vascular symptoms or colour change in arms? – thoracic outlet syndrome (TOS)
- Always ask about neck pain or stiffness

Injury history including mechanism of injury, in particular, any previous anterior shoulder dislocation or previous surgery?

Training history and occupation

- Sport played, volume and frequency of training
- Hand dominance
- If swimmer, what stroke and which side do they breathe on?
- Any recent changes in training volume?

Nutritional history

Rheumatological screen and include hypermobility screening questions

Systemic review and red flags

Past medical history (PMH)

Family history (FH)

Social history

Medications including supplements and over the counter (OTC) medications and allergies

Ideas, concerns and expectations (ICE)

Examination of the shoulder

Initial

- Wash hands
- Expose: Ensure shirt removed and in sports bra for females
- Ask patient to point to area of pain

Standing

- Inspection: Look from the front, the side and the back for global muscle bulk, scars and symmetry
- Global functional movement: Ask patient to put hands behind head (functional external rotation [ER]) or reach behind and touch back (internal rotation [IR])
- You could perform a cervical spine (C spine) screen at this point (cervical spine movement +/– Spurling's test if necessary)
- Palpate for bony tenderness and watch patient's face for pain
  - Sternoclavicular joint
  - Clavicle
  - Acromioclavicular joint (ACJ)

- Bicipital groove
- Acromion
- Scapular spine and medial and inferior borders
- Myofascial – trapezius, supraspinatus and infraspinatus
- Move: Active
  - Stand to the side and just behind patient so you can assess movement of scapulae but also see their face for pain
  - Ask the patient to move both arms up for forward flexion and compare both sides and then do the same for abduction
  - Perform passive ER with elbows tucked into side
  - IR: Ask the patient to slide their good arm up their spine as high as they can and compare it with their symptomatic side
  - If any reduction in active ROM, see if reduced passive ROM (in rotator cuff you get loss of active ROM but not passive ROM, whereas with adhesive capsulitis you get loss of both)
- Special tests (have one test, if positive then confirm with a second test)
  - Rotator cuff
    - Supraspinatus – Jobe's test (empty can in scapular plane with thumbs towards floor)
    - Infraspinatus/teres minor – resisted ER
    - Subscapularis – Gerber's lift off
  - The acronym BLISS can be used
    - Biceps – Speed and Yergason's tests
    - Labrum – O'Brien's test
    - Impingement – Hawkins Kennedy test
    - ACJ – Scarf test/adduction across body
    - Shoulder instability – inferior sulcus and anterior/posterior translation. Perform apprehension test in supine
  - Consider neural tension tests if indicated

Sitting

- Spurling's test (especially if reduced ROM or pain in cervical spine)
- Thoracic outlet tests
  - Roos test, Adson's test
- Neurological examination – tone, power, sensation, reflexes

Supine

- Special tests continued
  - Apprehension test for anterior instability
  - Posterior instability

Other

- Beighton score if instability (see the following box and Figure 2.1)

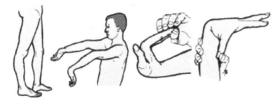

Figure 2.1 Tests for joint hypermobility include hyperextension of knees and elbows; metacarpophalangeal joints >90°; thumb able to touch forearm. (Reproduced with kind permission from *Apley & Solomon's System of Orthopaedics and Trauma*, 10th edition, CRC Press, 2018.)

The Beighton score consists of five manoeuvres

1. Passive opposition of thumb to forearm (left and right)
2. Passive hyperextension of little finger metacarpophalangeal joint >90° (left and right)
3. Active hyperextension of elbow >10° (left and right)
4. Active hyperextension of knee >10° (left and right)
5. Ability to flex spine placing palms to floor without bending knees

Each is worth 1 point and a score ≥4 out of 9 is positive.

Red flags

- Suspected infected joint
- Unreduced dislocation
- Suspected malignancy
- Acute rotator cuff tear
- Evidence of an underlying collagen disorder

Key points

- Always clear the C spine
- If instability, think is this part of a generalised hypermobility picture or post-traumatic?
- If global reduced ROM think adhesive capsulitis or osteoarthritis
- Rotator cuff tears have reduced active but preserved passive ROM

ELBOW

"Ralph is a 13-year-old cricketer who presents with a one-month history of elbow pain after a recent summer training camp. It is worst when he bowls and he has tried ice and paracetamol with little effect. Please take a focussed history and examination and present your differential diagnosis and management plan."

History

History of presenting complaint

- Onset of symptoms – acute injury or insidious onset?
- Pain – SOCRATES
- Site of pain is important in determining likely differentials (see Chapter 4)
  - Medial pain
  - Lateral pain
  - Posterior pain
- Any mechanical symptoms such as clicking or clunking? – loose body, osteochondral defect
- Any snapping sensation? – ulnar collateral ligament (UCL), accessory triceps
- Exacerbating activity or position
- Any features of hypermobility
- Always ask about neck pain or stiffness
- Neurological symptoms such as paraesthesia or weakness

Injury history including mechanism of injury (MOI)

Training history and occupation

- Dominant hand, sport played and volume of training
- Any recent changes in training volume?

Nutritional history

Rheumatological screen and include hypermobility screening questions

Systemic review and Red flags

Past medical history

Family history

Social history

Medications and allergies

ICE

Examination of the elbow

Initial

- Wash your hands
- Expose: Ensure patient is in minimum a T-shirt, or shirtless to assess shoulder
- Ask patient to point to the area of pain

Standing

- Inspection: Look from the front, the side and the back for global muscle bulk, scars and symmetry
- Hypermobility screen: Ask patient to extend elbows fully. If a wide carrying angle then perform a full Beighton score

- You could perform a shoulder and C spine screen at this point (shoulder abduction, IR and ER, C spine movement +/− Spurling's if necessary)
- Palpation
  - Medial – medial epicondyle, ulnar nerve
  - Lateral – lateral epicondyle, radial head, extensor muscle bulk
  - Anterior – biceps tendon
  - Posterior – olecranon
- Move: active— flexion, extension, pronation and supination (with elbows tucked in)
  - Passive: If any reduced active ROM
  - Resisted movement
- Special tests
  - Valgus stress (UCL)
  - UCL snapping with repeated flexion
  - Common extensor origin (CEO) tendinopathy - resisted wrist extension whilst palpating common flexor origin muscle bulk, resisted middle finger extension
  - Common flexor origin (CFO) tendinopathy - resisted wrist flexion whilst palpating common flexor origin muscle bulk
  - Tinel's test behind medial epicondyle
- End: Neurovascular examination including median, radial and ulnar examination and dermatomal examination

HAND AND WRIST

"A 52-year-old secretary has attended complaining of wrist and thumb pain bilaterally, worse at night. She has a BMI of 27 and is on a statin. Her General Practitioner (GP) has prescribed her some night splints but she is struggling to do her typing at work with her symptoms. Please assess."

In this scenario, you are told the symptoms are in the median nerve distribution. The focus should be on confirming this, and performing screening tests to rule out other regional differentials and peripheral nerve involvement.

History

History of presenting complaint

- Injury – MOI, e.g. fall onto an outstretched hand (FOOSH), rotational stress
- Pain – SOCRATES. Site of pain helps to differentiate:
  - Ulnar, radial, dorsal, volar
  - Night pain – carpal tunnel syndrome (CTS)
- Paraesthesia and distribution
- Clicking/instability – triangular fibrocartilage complex (TFCC) instability, extensor carpi ulnaris (ECU) subluxation, carpal bones
- Swelling – rule out systemic or rheumatological cause

- Stiffness – rule out rheumatological cause
- Deformity
- Loss of function
- Ask about neck pain or stiffness – C spine

Injury history including MOI

Training history and occupation

- Dominant hand, sport played and volume of training
- Any recent changes in training volume?
- Any recent unaccustomed exercise, e.g. gardening

Nutritional history

Rheumatological screen and include hypermobility screening questions

Systemic review and red flags

PMH: Diabetes mellitus, hypercholesterolaemia, chronic kidney disease (risk factors for carpal tunnel)

Family history

Social history including occupation and hobbies

Medications and allergies

ICE: How is this affecting their sport, daily life or occupation?

Examination of the hand and wrist

Initial

- Wash hands
- Expose patient above the elbows and place hands on a table or pillow on their lap
- Ask patient to indicate the area of pain

Inspection

- Posture of the hand, skin, swelling or muscle wasting
- Inspect the elbows for rheumatoid nodules and psoriasis plaques
- Deformities associated with rheumatoid arthritis – ulnar deviation, subluxation of metacarpal phalangeal joints (MCP)
- Fingers: Boutonniere, swan neck deformities or Z thumb deformity
- Nails: Onycholysis, clubbing

Functional movement

- Ask to make a fist, undo a button, pick up a coin

Feel

- Temperature using back of hand (synovitis)
- Palpation: Perform systematic palpation of the main structures starting with the dorsal aspect move radial to ulnar side (see Figure 2.2)

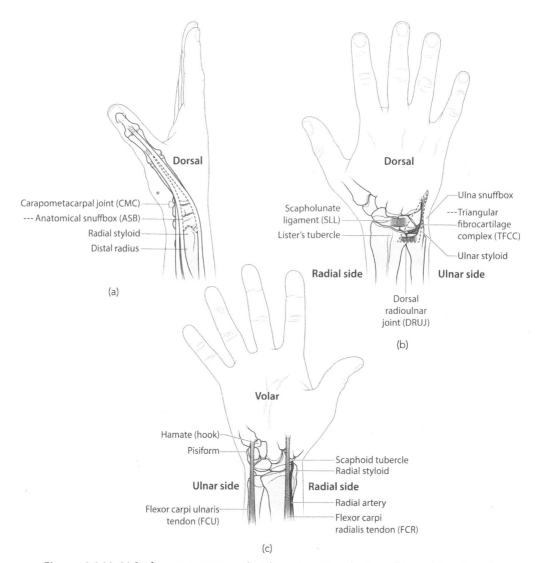

Figures 2.2 (a)–(c) Surface anatomy to undertake systematic palpation of the wrist and hand.

Wrist

Move: Active (and passive if not full active ROM)

- Wrist flexion and extension (prayer and reserve prayer to assess symmetry)
- Pronation and supination (with elbows flexed and tucked in)
- Radial and ulnar deviation (with hand flat on surface)

Resisted – wrist flexion, extension, pronation, supination and radial and ulnar deviation

Special tests if indicated:

- Pseudoinstability – lack of this indicates rigid capsule, pain or muscle spasm
- Scaphoid tubercle tenderness, snuffbox tenderness and pain on telescoping for scaphoid fracture
- Phalen and Tinel's test for carpal tunnel syndrome (CTS)
- Watson's test for scapholunate instability
- Finkelstein's test for De Quervain's tenosynovitis
- Piano key test for the distal radioulnar joint
- Froment's sign for ulnar nerve injury
- Ulnar collateral ligament stability for Gamekeeper's thumb
- Stress of triangular fibrocartilage complex – dorsiflex and ulnar deviate wrist

Fingers and thumb

Move:

- MCP, proximal interphalangeal joint (PIP) and distal interphalangeal joint (DIP) flexion and extension
- Thumb MCP and interphalangeal (IP) flexion and extension

Check finger flexion and extension of MCP, PIP and DIPs. In fist position fingers should point towards the scaphoid.

- Check interossei – abduction/adduction of fingers
- Check thumb movements
  - Abduction – median nerve
  - Adduction – ulnar nerve
  - Flexion, extension, opposition
- Check wrist grip strength – fist

Finish: Say you would like to examine the elbow and the C spine

Hand and wrist neurological examination

Peripheral nerves

1. **Median nerve (C5-T1)**
   - Potential sites of compression: Ligament of Struthers, pronator teres (anterior interosseous nerve [AIN]) or carpal tunnel syndrome
   - Inspection: Wasting of thenar eminence
   - Sensation: Tip of index finger, base of thenar eminence (normal in CTS)
   - Palpation: Thenar eminence muscle bulk
   - Motor testing
     - Abductor pollicis brevis (APB) – flex thumb towards ceiling
     - Opponens pollicis (OP) – press thumb and little finger together and resist being pulled apart
     - Anterior interosseous nerve (AIN) – flexor pollicis longus (FPL) and index flexor digitorum profundus (FDP) – ask to make 'OK' sign
   - Special tests: Tinel and Phalen's
   - Collection of clinical findings will be determined by the location of the medial nerve entrapment (Table 2.1)
2. **Radial nerve (C5-T1)**
   - Potential sites of compression: above the elbow, e.g. humeral spiral fracture, around the elbow (radial tunnel and posterior interosseous nerve [PIN]) and around the wrist
   - Inspection: Wrist drop
   - Sensation: 1st web space dorsum of hand (spared if posterior interosseous nerve)

- Palpation: Palpate the lateral elbow
- Motor testing:
  - Wrist extension
  - PIN:
    - Extensor Indicis (EI) – point with index finger
    - Extensor pollicis longus (EPL) – retropulsion of thumb with palm on table
    - Can extend wrist but deviates radially (extensor carpi ulnaris [ECU] affected)
- Special tests: Resisted active supination with elbow extended produces pain in PIN
- Note: Radial tunnel syndrome – pain but no weakness, PIN – pain and weakness
- High lesions will affect all muscles and there will be loss of sensation to the dorsum of thumb

3. **Ulnar nerve (C8, T1)**
   - Potential sites of compression: Cubital tunnel (affects intrinsic and extrinsic muscles), Guyon's canal (intrinsics only) (Table 2.2)
   - Inspection: Claw hand, interossei wasting, Wartenberg's sign (weak 3rd palmar interosseous), inspect the elbow
   - Sensation:
     - Palmar cutaneous branch innervates the medial half of the palm
     - Dorsal cutaneous branch innervated the dorsal surface of the medial one and a half fingers, and the associated dorsum of the hand
     - The superficial branch arises in the hand and innervates the palmar surface of the medial one and a half fingers.

   If a proximal lesion is present then sensation is reduced in both the dorsum of the 5th metacarpal (MC) and tip of little finger. If the lesion is in Guyon's canal, then there will be reduced sensation in the tip of little finger only.
   - Palpation: Cubital tunnel and Guyon's canal
   - Motor testing:
     - Extrinsics FCU and FDP of little and ring fingers – ask patient to 'tuck little

Table 2.1 Features of median nerve entrapment according to location

High lesion	Low lesion	Anterior interosseous nerve
• e.g. Entrapment at the elbow • Motor deficit • Thenar eminence sensory deficit	• e.g. Carpal tunnel syndrome • Flexor digitorum superficialis (FDS) and FCR preserved • Thenar eminence sensation preserved	• e.g. Entrapment at the tendinous edge of the deep head of pronator teres. • Pure motor deficit • Unable to perform 'OK' sign

Table 2.2 Features of ulnar nerve entrapment according to location

High lesion	Low lesion
• e.g. Medial epicondyle • Sensation in both areas lost • Motor: all muscles affected • Froment's sign + • Less clawing	• e.g. Guyon's canal • No loss of sensation in the dorsum 5th MC • Power of FDP little finger and FCU preserved • Pronounced clawing 'ulnar paradox'

finger into palm when you make a fist' (intact with low lesion)
  – Intrinsics – ask to cross fingers, press abducted little fingers together
• Special tests: Froment's sign, Tinel's test

Nerve roots/dermatomes

See Figure 2.3 and the section 'Neurological Examination' for details on nerve roots and dermatomes.

Sensation

    C6 – thumb pad
    C7 – middle finger pad
    C8 – little finger pad

Power

    C5 – elbow flexion
    C6 – wrist extensors
    C7 – triceps extension
    C8 – finger flexion
    T1 – finger abductors

Reflexes

    Biceps   – C5
    Brachioradialis – C6
    Triceps   – C7

Spurling's test

LUMBAR SPINE

George is a 16-year-old gymnast who has been referred by his GP with a 3-month history of lower back pain. His pain is worse on landing and when arching his back but not at rest. He has no significant past medical history. He has no other joint problems and takes paracetamol and ibuprofen if the pain is particularly bad. Please take a history and focussed examination and present your findings.

History

History of presenting complaint

• Onset of symptoms – acute injury or insidious
• Pain – SOCRATES
  • Site
  • Onset
  • Character
  • Radiation
  • Associations
  • Time course
  • Exacerbating/Relieving Factors
  • Severity – scale 1–10
• Is the pain during or after exercise or at rest/at night?
• Whether pain is flexion or extension related
• Any neurological symptoms – leg weakness, paraesthesia
• Whether any treatment has been used, e.g. analgesia or physiotherapy and whether this has helped

Training history

Gymnast

• Discipline performed, e.g. floor, bar
• Any recent change in load? E.g. volume, duration or intensity of training sessions or reduction in rest periods

Cricket

• Position played, e.g. *fast bowler or spin?*
• Any change in volume or intensity of training – *How many overs does he bowl per year?*
• Current level played and aims for the season

Nutritional history

• Do they keep a diet diary and its relation to training?
• Are there any features of RED-S? *oligomenorrhoea (if female), fatigue, regular infections, underperformance, previous stress fractures, poor sleep*

It is essential to ask questions to screen for an underlying rheumatological diagnosis:

• Morning stiffness >1 hour, history of psoriasis, history of inflammatory bowel disease, Achilles tendon inflammation, anterior uveitis (ask about red, painful eyes), strong family history, any urinary symptoms or diarrhoea (reactive arthritis such as gonococcal or campylobacter infection). It may be appropriate to explore a sexual history if so

Systemic review

• Weight loss, fever, night sweats – *consider sinister causes, e.g. spinal TB, malignancy*

Specifically ask about red flags

• Any symptoms of cauda equina, e.g. bladder bowel disturbance, leg weakness, saddle anaesthesia
• Weight loss
• Night pain
• Altered bladder/bowel function, e.g. urinary retention

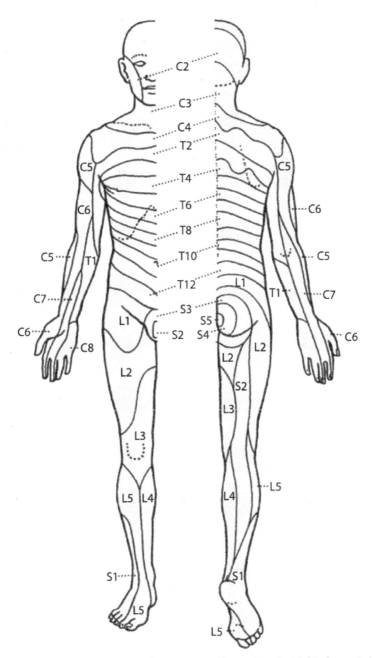

Figure 2.3 Dermatomes supplied by the spinal nerve roots. (Reproduced with kind permission from *Apley & Solomon's System of Orthopaedics and Trauma*, 10th edition, CRC Press, 2018.)

- Bilateral lower leg weakness
- PMH cancer
- Fever
- Prolonged use of corticosteroids

Past medical history – including previous injuries, history of osteoporosis, prior eating disorder

Family history – Do rheumatological conditions run in the family?

Social history

Medication history and allergies – including supplements and OTC medications

ICE – How is this impacting their life and training? What is the patient worried about?

Examination of the lumbar spine

To look slick, you don't want to be making the patient go from standing to sitting to lying to prone multiple times and so the following recommended examination order allows you to perform a smooth examination with a logical sequence of manoeuvres. You can say out loud 'I would now like to perform a neurological screening test' – the examiner may state this is normal and ask you to move on to save time. If you anticipate it to be normal, it is still important to state it to demonstrate you recognise the need to perform a neurological screen in all patients with back pain.

Recommended order of focussed examination in 7–8 minutes for a 10-minute station, plus questions.

Initial

- Wash your hands
- Expose: Ensure patient is in shorts and bare feet and that you can visualise the lumbar spine (shirtless for males and in sports bra for females)
- Ask patient to point to indicate the area of their pain or symptoms

Standing

Inspection:

- Look from the front, side and back of the patient for global muscle bulk and alignment/posture. *If wide carrying angle of elbows or genu recurvatum noted, incorporate full Beighton score into assessment.*
- Assess gait: Ask the patient to walk to the end of the room, turn around and walk back to you. *Squat down and make a comment on what you see, e.g. 'this patient has a non-antalgic gait with normal alignment of the pelvis, knee and foot.'*
- Perform 1–2 relevant functional tests:
  - Double leg squat then single leg squat – *comment on lumbopelvic stability, look for medial knee drift*
  - Hop test

Move

- Ask patient to perform lumbar flexion, extension and lateral flexion whilst inspecting from behind – *here you can comment on lumbar lordosis or any restriction in movement. If lumbar flexion appears restricted say you would perform a Schober's test*
- Perform Stork test or quadrant test – *a positive test would indicate posterolateral structure pathology, e.g. pars or facet joint*
- Neurological screen – perform gross motor neurology screen – ask patient to squat (L3), walk on heels (L4), lift hallux up (L5), stand on tiptoes (S1)

Sitting

- Perform slump test on edge of couch
- Perform Thomas' test – *hip flexion indicates tight iliopsoas, knee extension indicates tight rectus femoris, lateral drift of leg indicates tight Iliotibial band (ITB)*

Supine

- Screen the hip:

- Passive movement: Hip flexion, internal and external rotation, abduction and adduction – comment on range of movement or if painful
- Perform flexion, adductor, IR (FADIR) and flexion, abduction and ER (FABER)
- Say you would perform a lower limb neurological exam (see the following box and the section 'Neurological examination') – *the examiner may move you on*

Lower limb neurological examination findings according to nerve root affected

Sensation	Muscle power	Reflexes
L3 – Inside knee	Knee extension	Knee (L3,4)
L4 – Inside ankle	Ankle dorsiflexion	
L5 – 1st web space	Dorsiflexion of the first toe	Ankle (L5,S1)
S1 – Heel	Plantar flexion of the ankle and toes	

- Screen the SIJ:
  - Perform Laslett's sacroiliac joint (SIJ) tests (the following sequence moves the patient from supine to prone smoothly) (1): (1) thigh thrust (supine), (2) side compression (on their side), (3) distraction (prone), (4) compression (prone)

Prone

- Inspection – *comment on any muscle wasting, scars or asymmetry*
- Palpation
  - Using heel of hand palpate SIJ and spinous processes for pain or step deformity, moving distal to proximal
  - After each spinous process, palpate lateral structures on both sides (facet/pars/transverse process)
  - Paraspinal and gluteal muscles for increased tone or trigger points

To conclude

- Thank the patient
- Say you would also like to examine the thoracic spine and perform a per rectum (PR) exam if indicated
- Depending on the findings, e.g. restricted lumbar flexion and lateral flexion indicating possible seronegative disease say you would like to look for other features of seronegative

disease by assessing the eyes for anterior uveitis and the Achilles for enthesitis and would also like to perform a Schober's test

Things to avoid

- Illogical sequence of examination requiring patient to stand and sit multiple times
- Causing pain to the patient
- Failing to screen the hip or SIJ
- Failing to at least state you would do a neurological exam
- Neglecting to exclude red flags or underlying rheumatological diagnosis
- Omitting a training history which may indicate load-related injury

HIP AND GROIN

"Paul is a 35-year-old office worker who has been referred by his GP with a 4-month history of hip pain. George is a keen amateur runner and is a member of his local running group, accruing an average of 100km per week road running. His pain is worse after a long run. He has no significant past medical history. Please take a history and focussed examination and present your findings."

History

History of presenting complaint

- Onset of symptoms – acute injury or insidious
- Hip pain using SOCRATES.
- Hip pain location is important to establish.
  - Lateral pain may indicate a gluteus medius tendinopathy or greater trochanteric pain syndrome (GTPS) whilst when some patients describe 'hip' pain they actually point to posterior/buttock pain which could be referred from the lumbar spine or SIJ
  - Iliopsoas injury is normally felt as groin or proximal thigh pain
  - Adductor injury is felt in the groin/pubis
- Groin pain may be present in athletes with a traction apophysis
- Mechanical symptoms, e.g. locking, clicking – suspect labral pathology or snapping hip syndrome
- Ask about back pain or neurological symptoms
- Any urinary symptoms or genitourinary problems?

Past medical history: Ask about previous developmental problems with hips as a child or adolescent, menstrual history

Family history

Social history

Drug history: ask about steroids

Training and nutrition history – especially important if you suspect a stress fracture in a runner

ICE

Examination of the hip and groin

Initial

- Wash your hands and ask patient to point to the area of pain
- Expose: Ensure patient is in shorts and bare feet and that you can adequately visualise the lumbar spine (shirtless for males and in sports bra for females)

Standing

- Inspection: Look at the general posture of the patient, any asymmetry in the anterior superior iliac spine (ASIS) on either side and any obvious muscle wasting
- Assess gait: Ask the patient to walk to the end of the room, turn around and walk back to you. Squat down and make a comment on what you see, e.g. *'this patient has a non-antalgic gait with normal alignment of the pelvis, knee and foot.'*
- Perform 1–2 functional tests:
  - Double leg squat then single leg squat – comment on lumbopelvic stability
  - Hop test – if positive for pain, consider a femoral neck stress fracture
  - Trendelenberg test
- Screen lumbar spine in standing: Lumbar flexion, extension and lateral flexion – here you can comment on lumbar lordosis
  - Stork test or quadrant test to assess posterior elements

Sitting

- Perform slump test on the edge of the couch
- Perform Thomas' test - *hip flexion indicates tight iliopsoas, knee extension indicates tight rectus femoris, lateral drift of leg indicates tight Iliotibial band (ITB)*

Supine

- Palpation – ASIS, anterior inferior iliac spine (AIIS), anterior hip joint, inguinal ligament, pubic symphysis, adductors, greater trochanter, glute medius and minimum tendons and muscle belly (this can also be done with patient lying on their side)

Movement

- Passive movement: Hip flexion (120°), internal (40°) and external rotation (45°), abduction (45°) and adduction (30°)
  - Comment on range of movement or if painful

Table 2.3 Adductor squeeze test and corresponding muscles

Knees extended	Adductor magnus and gracilis
Knees 45°	Adductor longus and pubic joint
Knees 90°	Pectineus and abdominals

- Resisted movement – flexion, extension, abduction and adduction

Special tests whilst supine .

- FADIR test for femoroacetabular impingement (FAI)
- Quadrant test for an intraarticular lesion
- FABER test – a positive test may indicate pathology in the SIJ, hip or spine
- Adductor squeeze test (fist between knees with legs extended, at 45° and at 90°; see Table 2.3)
- Perform a full screen of the SIJ

KNEE

"A 17-year-old volleyball player has presented to your clinic with a two week history of knee pain. They describe pain just below their kneecap which is worse on jumping and came on after a recent training camp. There is no clicking or clunking and no obvious swelling. Please take a history and focussed examination and present your findings."

History

History of presenting complaint

- Mechanism of injury – cutting or pivoting movement? – think anterior cruciate injury (ACL)
- Pain – SOCRATES
  - Anterior knee pain – patellofemoral joint (PFJ), patellar tendon
    - What particular exacerbates their pain? Jumping? Prolonged sitting?
  - Medial vs lateral structures
  - Posterior knee pain
  - Vague pain – patellofemoral joint, ACL, osteoarthritis
  - Is there any hip pain, especially if paediatric or adolescent patient?
- Swelling – presence of absence, was it immediate or did it appear the following day?
  - Haemarthrosis – ACL injury, osteochondral lesion, patellar dislocation
  - Delayed – meniscal tear, some ACL tears
- Did they hear a 'pop' – ACL or patellar dislocation
- Mechanical symptoms – loose body or meniscal tear or giving way (giving way generally indicates instability)
- Treatment history

Past medical history

Injury history – Any previous knee injuries or surgeries? What is their level of sport played and position? Which leg do they kick a ball with?

Training and nutritional history

Drug history

Social – occupation

ICE

Examination of the knee

Initial

- Wash hands
- Expose patient – in shorts with no shoes or socks on
- Ask patient to point to area of pain

Standing

- Inspection – look from the front, the side and from behind
  - Comment on genu recurvatum and global alignment
  - Gait – ask patient to walk up and down (squat down when inspecting gait)
  - Comment if gait antalgic or not, assess alignment of pelvis, knee and foot and ankle
- Perform functional movement
  - Ask patient to squat with feet flat on the floor and assess for ROM or quality of movement (if heels lift off the floor, there may either be pain or posterior chain tightness)
  - Ask to squat down with heels up to assess the posterior meniscus
  - Duck walk – meniscal screen
  - Single leg squat – assess for pelvic drop or knee valgus indicating poor proximal control
  - Hop test – if positive the possible differentials may include anterior knee pain, tendinopathy or stress fracture
  - Thessaly test for meniscal screen

Supine: With knee extended

- Local Inspection – comment on skin changes, scars of previous surgery or swelling
- Assess for an effusion
  - Large effusion – Patellar tap
  - Small effusion – sweep test and assess for medial fluid collection
- Move – assess flexion ROM (should be 140°) and extension ROM (normally hyperextension to 0° to −5°)

Supine: With knee flexed

- Palpate
  - Palpate anterior, middle and posterior lateral joint line and fibula

- Medial joint line, medial collateral ligament (MCL) and pes anserinus insertion
- Tibial tuberosity
- Distal, medial and proximal patellar tendon/inferior pole of patella
- Posterior knee
- Palpate fad pad either side of tendon and extend knee (fat pad impingement)

Supine: With knee extended

- Patellar and PFJ assessment
  - Palpate under patellar on lateral and medial sides for pain
  - Clark's test for PFJ
  - Lateral glide for apprehension

Special tests

- Check for sag sign with both knees flexed for posterior cruciate ligament integrity (PCL)
- Assess both collateral ligaments in extension and 30° flexion
- Anterior drawer test and Lachman's test for ACL +/− pivot shift
- McMurray's test for menisci

Supine: Consider if appropriate

Supine: Lateral – Ober's test for ITB
Prone: Apley's grind (meniscal injury) and dial test (PCL injury if >10°)

At the end

State you would examine the joint above and below.

HAMSTRING

"A 23-year-old footballer has presented the morning after a match with a "tight right hamstring". He can't remember a particular incident or injury but had a sore right hamstring immediately after the game when he was cooling down. He reports no neurological symptoms. Please assess."

History

History of presenting complaint

- Mechanism of injury. Was it during sudden muscle contraction or slow stretch?
- Could they immediately weight bear after? – good prognosis
- SOCRATES
  - What is the exact location of pain?
  - Proximal vs distal?
  - Is this referred from SIJ?
- Is there any associated back pain?
- Any neurological symptoms such as weakness or paraesthesia?

Past medical history

Injury history – Is this recurrent? What has their management been since they sustained the injury?

Training and nutritional history

Drug history

Social – occupation

ICE

Examination

Standing

- Inspection – any visible ecchymosis, swelling or difference in muscle bulk?
- Gait – antalgic
- Functional tests
  - Assess trunk flexion with hands touching legs – can they reach to knees, mid-shins, ankles or floor?
  - Double leg squat to 90°
  - Single leg squat to 45°
  - Lunge
- Screen the lumbar spine as symptoms could be referred

Sitting

- Slump test to rule out L5/S1 radiculopathy
- Modified Thomas' test

Supine

- Screen the hip and knee
- Ask the patient to perform a double leg bridge, then single leg bridge to assess for pain and lumbopelvic stability
- Assess passive straight leg raise
- Assess degree of knee extension with hip flexed to 90° and at maximal flexion
- Thigh thrust for SIJ

Prone

- Identify the most painful area and measure the distance from the ischial tuberosity
- Palpate the ischial tuberosity, biceps femoris, semimembranosus and semitendinosus
- Palpate the gluteal muscles
- Test resisted hip extension and knee flexion
- Complete SIJ screening

Additional: Can assess isometric strength of knee flexion whilst prone

CALF

"A 40-year-old businessman has presented to Accident and Emergency (A&E) unable to weight bear after feeling a 'pop' in the back of his leg playing squash. He has had no significant previous injuries and currently takes a statin for high cholesterol. Please take a focussed history and examination."

History

History of presenting complaint

- Mechanism of injury – was it sudden or did symptoms come on insidiously?
- Could they immediately weight bear after?
- Did they hear a 'pop'? (Achilles rupture)
- SOCRATES
  - What is the exact location of pain?
  - Proximal vs distal?
  - Localised vs diffuse pain
- Is there any knee, hip or back pain?
- Any neurological symptoms such as weakness or paraesthesia?
- Any recent long distance travel or immobilisation (DVT)?

Past medical history

Injury history – is this recurrent? What has their management been since they sustained the injury?

Training and nutritional history

Drug history

Social – occupation

ICE

Examination

Standing

- Inspection – muscle bulk, biomechanical abnormalities
- Gait – assess for antalgic gait
- Ask to perform a knee to wall test and compare distance of the wall to the tip of the big toe using a tape measure
- Functional tests
  - Double leg squat
  - Single leg squat
  - Jump
  - Single leg calf raise to fatigue

Prone

- Palpate along medial and lateral gastrocnemius and soleus for area of maximal tenderness
- Assess knee and ankle passive ROM
- Resisted ankle movements – does plantarflexion cause pain?
- Palpate Achilles tendon for any discontinuity
- Perform Simmond's test

LEG PAIN

"An 18-year-old infantryman presents complaining of bilateral "shin pain" which came on 2 weeks after starting his basic training. It is worse when running. An X-ray was performed which is normal. He has no significant past medical history. Please assess."

History

History of presenting complaint

- Location of pain
- Is the pain bilateral or unilateral?
- Is there a history of increased load especially running, tabbing, walking fast or uphill?
- Has there been a change in equipment, shoes, training or conditions?
- Onset and duration of pain
  - Does pain 'warm up': medial tibial stress syndrome (MTSS) or tendinopathy
  - Rest pain: stress fracture, red flag
  - Pain ceases after activity: chronic exertional compartment syndrome (CECS), popliteal artery entrapment
  - Creschendo 'bursting pain': CECS
- Muscle herniation: CECS
- Sensory symptoms, e.g. pins and needles: nerve entrapment or CECS

Past medical history – ask about peripheral vascular disease

Injury history – is this recurrent?

Training and nutritional history

Drug history

Social – occupation

ICE

Examination

Standing

- Inspection
- Gait – are there any obvious biomechanical abnormalities e.g. pes planus?
- Functional movement
  - Single leg stand and single leg squat
  - Knee to wall distance
  - Gastrocnemius stretch against wall – comment on if any obvious herniations
  - Heel raises – how many can they perform on each side?

Sitting

- Slump test or SLR

Get supine

- Passive knee ROM
- Ankle passive ROM
- Ankle resisted movements
- Palpate area of tenderness i.e. pinpoint bony tenderness, diffuse? or soft tissue
  - Palpate entire tibia and fibula
  - Percussive tenderness – pain if stress fracture, if reproduces neuropathic symptoms consider peripheral nerve entrapment, could use tuning fork

- Often tight and weak posterior chain
- Check pulses however unlikely to be reduced at rest unless severe stenosis

Prone

- Feel calf and assess tightness in soleus and gastrocnemius – straight knee vs bent knee

Closing: Say you would like to examine the hip and knee and potentially re-examine after activity to exacerbate symptoms

FOOT AND ANKLE

"A 35-year-old office worker presents complaining of pain in her heel which came on after a long walk over the weekend. She describes it as "aching" and is worse when weight bearing. Please assess."

History

History of presenting complaint

- Onset of symptoms – acute injury or insidious
- Pain – SOCRATES
  - Site – anterior, posterior, lateral or medial?
  - Onset
  - Character
  - Radiation
  - Associations
  - Time course
  - Exacerbating/relieving factors
  - Severity – scale 1–10
- Is the pain during or after exercise or at rest/ at night? Is there morning stiffness/takes time to warm up (Achilles tendinopathy or seronegative disease)?
- Is the ankle joint stiff?
- Any neurological symptoms – leg weakness, paraesthesia
- Ask about footwear/any change in footwear

Injury history – is this recurrent? What has their management been since they sustained the injury?

Training and nutritional history

Drug history

Social – occupation

ICE

Examination of the foot and ankle

Initial

- Wash hands
- Expose patient – in shorts with no shoes or socks on
- Ask patient to point to area of pain

Standing

- Inspection – look from the front, the side and from behind

- Comment on the medial arch, pes planus, too many toes sign
- Gait – ask patient to walk up and down (squat down when inspecting gait)
  - Comment if gait antalgic or not, assess alignment of pelvis, knee and foot and ankle
- Perform functional movement
  - Squat
  - Single leg squat
  - One legged balance – proprioception
  - Heel raises to fatigue
  - Hop test
  - From behind ask them to go onto tiptoes to assess for normal varus position of heel (suggests tibialis posterior tendon is intact)

Supine

Get them to bend their knee and place the sole of their foot on the bed.

- Palpate
  - Lateral: Base of 5th metatarsal (MT), fibula (entire length), lateral ligaments in turn and sinus tarsi
  - Anterior – squeeze test for syndesmosis, palpate the talus
  - Medial – medial malleolus, behind medial malleolus for flexor hallucis longus (FHL) and tibialis posterior, navicular and deltoid ligament
- Move (get them to extend their knee)
  - Active – dorsiflexion/plantarflexion, inversion/eversion
  - Passive – subtalar ROM, midtarsal ROM
  - Resisted dorsiflexion/plantarflexion, plantarflexion of hallux, inversion/eversion, resisted hallux plantarflexion (FHL)
- Special tests
  - Squeeze test and ER test for syndesmosis injury
  - Anterior drawer test (anterior talofibular ligament [ATFL] injury)
  - Tinel's test behind medial malleolus
  - Anterior and posterior impingement tests

Prone

- Inspection
  - Normal plantarflexed posture of foot indicates the Achilles tendon is intact
  - Any obvious thickening of Achilles tendon or swelling
- Palpate
  - Length of Achilles tendon for palpable defect, thickening +/– crepitus, plantar fascia insertion and along the plantar fascia, along the length of FHL and tibialis posterior, heel squeeze (calcaneus fracture) and sesamoids if local pain
  - Soleus and gastrocnemius

- Special tests
  - Simmonds test for Achilles tendon, extend the hallux for Windlass mechanism and observe the medial arch

Other

- Complete by saying you would examine the knee, spine and inspect shoes and perform a lower limb neurovascular examination
- If enthesopathy say you would like to examine for other features of seronegative disease e.g. eye examination, lumbar spine examination and urine dip for glucose in diabetes mellitus (DM)

NEUROLOGICAL EXAMINATION

It is perfectly reasonable that you may get a station where a patient has had a head injury and they require a cranial nerve examination. If this is the case, think about the mechanism of injury to focus your examination on the particular cranial nerves that are more likely to be affected e.g. eye movements if zygomatic complex injury.

Cranial nerve examination

I. Olfactory

II. Optic

III. Oculomotor

IV. Trochlear

V. Trigeminal

VI. Abducens

VII. Facial

VIII. Vestibulocochlear

IX. Glossopharyngeal

X. Vagus

XI. Spinal accessory

XII. Hypoglossal

a. Eyes (II, III, IV, VI)
- General – inspect patient's face and eyes
- Acuity – formally assess with Snellen chart or count fingers
- Fields
- Pupils – size and outline, direct and indirect light reflex, swinging light test, accommodation
- Movements – check for nystagmus or diplopia
- Fundi

b. Face (V,VII)
- Trigeminal nerve (V)
- Motor
  - Inspect for wasting of temporalis, ask patient to clench teeth (feel masseter and temporalis muscles), resisted jaw opening
  - Jaw jerk
- Sensory
  - V1 – forehead
  - V2- cheek
  - V3 – lower lip
  - Corneal reflex
- Facial nerve (VII)
  - Inspect for symmetry
  - Ask patient to show you their teeth and close eyes tightly – test strength of orbicularis oculi
  - Ask the patient to raise their eyebrows

c. Vestibulocochlear (VIII)
- Auditory
  - Rub fingers together next to each ear with other ear blocked
  - Rinne's and Weber's test
- Vestibular
  - Ataxia, inability to do heel-toe walk
  - Nystagmus

d. Mouth and tongue (IX, X, XII)
- Mouth and tongue
  - Ask patient to open mouth and inspect the tongue. Ask to protrude the tongue and look for deviation. Test strength of tongue by asking them to push the tongue on the side of their cheek and test power
- Pharynx
  - Inspect position of uvula and ask patient to say 'ahh,' assess swallow and gag reflex
- Larynx
  - Assess quality of cough
  - Assess speech volume and quality

e. Neck – accessory nerve (XI)
- Inspect neck and shoulders – sternocleidomastoid wasting/fasciculation
- Test sternocleidomastoid – ask patient to turn head to one side and push against forehead
- Test trapezius by getting patient to shrug against resistance

Upper limb neurological examination

Inspection – look at patient's shoulder and arm posture and any evidence of scars

Assess tone of the upper limbs

Sensation –

C5 – Deltoid/regimental badge

C6 – thumb pad

C7 – middle finger pad

C8 – little finger pad

T1 – medial elbow. Assess for Horner's syndrome

Table 2.4 A summary of symptoms and signs to specifically ask about in the history as part of a systems review

System	Symptoms
Cardiovascular	Chest pain, palpitations, syncope, dyspnoea, ankle oedema, orthopnoea, paroxysmal nocturnal dyspnoea
Respiratory	Dyspnoea, wheeze, cough, stridor, haemoptysis
Gastrointestinal	Nausea, vomiting, diarrhoea, abdominal pain, heartburn, change in bowel habit, blood/mucus in stool, weight loss, anorexia, jaundice, haematemasis
Neurological	Fits/faints/falls, headache, dizziness, vision, memory loss, neck stiffness, photophobia, seizures, paraesthesia
Endocrine	Polyuria, polydipsia, fatigue
Rheumatological	Arthralgia, swollen joints, morning stiffness >1 hour, uveitis, enthesitis
GUM	Urinary frequency, urgency, discharge, dysuria, haematuria, rash
B symptoms	Weight loss, fever, night sweats, lymphadenopathy
GUM, genitourinary medicine.	

Power – Grade on a scale of 0–5 on Medical Research Council's (MRC) muscle power scale (see the following box)

Muscle power grading using the Medical Research Council (MRC) scale

0 No contraction
1 Flick or trace of contraction
2 Active movement, with gravity eliminated
3 Active movement against gravity
4 Active movement against gravity and resistance
5 Normal power

C5 – Elbow flexion
C6 – Wrist extensors
C7 – Elbow extension
C8 – Finger flexion
T1 – Finger abductors

Reflexes

C5 – Biceps
C6 – Brachioradialis
C7 – Triceps

Coordination using finger to nose testing (if relevant)

Neural tension tests

Spurling's test for cervical radiculopathy (in sequence): Cervical extension followed by rotation of the head then finally axial compression. If there is a suggestion of cervical spine involvement than cervical movement should be assessed and a lower limb examination performed

Peripheral nerve examination of the hand and wrist is covered in the section 'Hand and wrist'

Lower limb neurological examination

Gait

Inspection

Assess tone of the lower limbs including clonus and Babinski

Sensation

L3 – Medial knee
L4 – Medial ankle
L5 – 1st web space
S1 – Heel

Power

L1/2 – Hip flexion
L3   – Knee extension
L4   – Ankle dorsiflexion
L5   – Dorsiflexion of the first toe
S1   – Ankle plantar flexion

Reflexes

L3/4 – Knee jerk
L5/S1 – Ankle

Peripheral nerves of the lower limb

SYSTEMS REVIEW

You may get a station where an athlete presents with a medical complaint, e.g. shortness of breath, abdominal pain, dizziness. You should be diligent in covering a systems review to consider the wider differentials and rule out red flags. Some of the key things you should cover in the history according to system are outlined in Table 2.4.

REFERENCE

1. Laslett M, et al. Diagnosis of sacroiliac joint pain: Validity of individual provocation tests and composites of tests. *Man Ther.* 2005;10(3):207–18.

Clinical cases

INTRODUCTION

Clinical cases in sport and exercise medicine objective structured clinical examinations (OSCEs) are a fundamental assessment of bedside manner and diagnostic acumen. The spectrum of clinical cases may be tested by stations predominantly consisting of history taking, examination or, more often, a combination of both. The marking scheme will depend upon the exact exam you are sitting and which institution, but it will normally assess various aspects of your performance in the following areas:

- Physical examination
- Identifying clinical signs
- Differential diagnosis
- Clinical judgement
- Managing patient concerns
- Maintaining patient welfare

There will be an objective marking criteria, and any follow-up questions have usually been standardised.

The following chapters are by no means exhaustive of all of the possible differentials that could come up in a clinical station in a sport and exercise medicine OSCE but covers the key points for the main diagnoses. Important differential diagnoses have been listed for each joint. For several of the diagnoses, a short clinical vignette has been described in italics. In the exam, there may be a similar introduction to read before you start the station. Use this time wisely to carefully read what information they have provided and start to formulate a plan for when you enter the station. Some stations may be more history focussed, others will want a focussed history and examination followed by a discussion. It should be clear from the instructions beforehand what is required of you. Although not covered extensively in this book, the reader should also be aware of acute fractures and their investigations and management which can be found in most comprehensive trauma and orthopaedic or emergency medicine texts.

DOI: 10.1201/9781003163701-4

3 Shoulder and upper limb

KEY DIFFERENTIAL DIAGNOSES OF THE SHOULDER

- Labral injury
- Rotator cuff injury
- Shoulder instability
- Capsular pain – including adhesive capsulitis
- Osteoarthritis
- Acromioclavicular joint (ACJ) injury
- Referred pain – cervical spine, myofascial, thoracic outlet

SUPERIOR LABRAL ANTERIOR TO POSTERIOR (SLAP) TEAR

"This right-handed 22-year-old tennis player presents with an insidious onset of shoulder pain provoked by serving and feels their serve is becoming weaker. Please assess."

A SLAP tear is an injury of the glenoid labrum. SLAP refers to superior labrum anterior to posterior and may or may not have long head of biceps involvement.

Mechanism of injury: Repetitive overhead activities or a sudden, acute event

Clinical features:

- 'Pop' during overhead activities or trauma
- Vague, deep shoulder pain
- Mechanical symptoms, e.g. clicking or clunking
- Easy fatigue

Signs:

- Bicipital groove tenderness
- Special tests: Speed's test +, Yergason's test +, O-Brien's test +
- Glenohumeral internal rotation deficit (GIRD)

Investigations:

- Magnetic resonance imaging (MRI) labral sequences +/– arthrogram

- MR arthrogram would demonstrate high signal (fluid on T2-weighted image [T2WI]) extending and tracking into the superior labrum +/– biceps (see Chapter 18)

Classification: Snyder classification (1)

Type I: Labral and biceps fraying
Type II: Labral fraying with detached biceps tendon anchor
Type III: Bucket handle tear with intact biceps anchor
Type IV: Bucket handle tear with detached biceps

Management:

1. Rehabilitation normally first line – Phased progressive programme
   a. Acute phase – Activity modification, education and analgesia.
   b. Subacute phase – Exercise should consist of rotator cuff exercises and scapular exercises with progressive load and complexity and stretching, e.g. cross-body or sleeper stretch. Initially protect biceps in early rehabilitation. Later exercises should link with kinetic chain.
   c. Sport-specific phase should include dynamic exercises using whole kinetic chain and gradually aiming to restore full velocity overhead movements, e.g. serving.
2. Operative management indicated if failed conservative management with severe symptoms or traumatic injuries with structural damage. Surgery depends on the type of lesion and biceps involvement; arthroscopic debridement considered for types I, III and IV tears involving <1/3 biceps tendon whilst a repair is indicated for Type IV tears with >1/3 of biceps involvement.

DOI: 10.1201/9781003163701-5

ROTATOR CUFF INJURY

Injuries to the rotator cuff can either be chronic degenerative, chronic impingement (of the rotator cuff muscles between the greater tuberosity of the humerus and acromion, coracoid or coracoacromial ligament) or an acute injury.

Symptoms:

- Pain on overhead activities
- Deltoid pain
- Night pain
- Weakness

Signs: Loss of active range of movement (ROM) with intact passive ROM. Special tests will be positive with corresponding muscle involvement:

- Supraspinatus: Jobe/empty can test +
- Infraspinatus/Teres minor: Pain on resisted external rotation (ER)
- Subscapularis: Gerber's lift off or belly press test +

Investigations:

- Ultrasound (US) may show hypoechoic defects in the tendon, fluid along the biceps tendon or an effusion in the subacromial/subdeltoid bursa or the glenohumeral joint. Indirect signs include a bright aspect of the humeral cartilage (cartilage interface sign). A full thickness tear is indicated by a defect that reaches from the bursal to the articular margin.
- MRI may show a defect in the tendon filled with fluid in T2, tendon retraction +/− subdeltoid bursal effusion or fluid along the biceps (see Chapter 18). Muscle atrophy and fatty replacement can be seen in chronic cases.

Classification: Ellman classification (see the following box) which was originally described in the supraspinatus. Injuries can be articular, bursal or interstitial/intratendinous (Figure 3.1). Most injuries are articular sided which are common in athletes participating in overhead activities.

Ellman classification (2)

Location	Grade
A: Articular surface	I: <3 mm (<25%)
B: Bursal surface	II: 3–6 mm (25–50%)
C: Interstitial	III: >6 mm (>50%)

Management:

1. Progressive rehabilitation focussing on specific rotator cuff strengthening following the acute phase, then conditioning and sport-specific graded return to play
2. Surgical options such as debridement or repair will depend on the patient (age and activity level) and the grade and type of tear. A rotator cuff repair may be offered in the following cases:
   a. An acute full-thickness tear in a young overhead athlete
   b. Bursal-sided tears >25%
   c. Partial articular-sided tears <50%

Surgical opinion can be sought in those who have failed conservative management.

SHOULDER IMPINGEMENT

Shoulder impingement represents a spectrum of pathology from subacromial bursitis to rotator cuff tendinopathy and cuff tears. It describes the entrapment of the rotator cuff muscles between the greater tuberosity of the humerus and acromion, coracoid or coracoacromial ligament. It can refer to either bony impingement, functional impingement due to muscle imbalance and poor scapulohumeral control, or intratendinous changes.

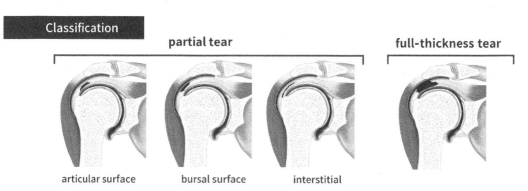

Classification

partial tear **full-thickness tear**

articular surface bursal surface interstitial

Figure 3.1 Partial tears can either be articular (on the side of the humerus; most common), bursal (on the side of the subacromial bursa) or intratendinous (interstitial). Full-thickness tears reach from the bursal to the articular margin.

Subacromial impingement: Subacromial impingement is the most common and tends to involve the entrapment of supraspinatus in the subacromial space (space between the acromion and the coracoid process and the coracoacromial ligament).

Symptoms: Insidious onset of pain lifting objects overhead or away from the body

Signs:

- Painful arc in 60–120° of flexion
- Neer test +
- Hawkins Kennedy test +
- Jobe test +

Subcoracoid impingement: Subcoracoid impingement is the entrapment of subscapularis between the coracoid and lesser tuberosity. It is less common than subacromial impingement.

Symptoms: Shoulder pain worsened by elevation and internal rotation or abduction.

Signs:

- Painful arc in 120–130° of flexion
- Pain on palpation of the lateral coracoid process
- Yokum test +

Investigations for impingement:

- Diagnosis can be clinical
- Imaging can support the diagnosis:
  - X-rays (anterior posterior (AP) and axillary views) can detect anatomical variants, calcification or osteoarthritis
  - US or MRI can help identify partial- or full-thickness tears and assess the bursa

Management:

- Depends on the individual case and activity levels of the patient.
- Conservative management is first line, including activity modification, analgesia, physiotherapy and consideration of a corticosteroid subacromial injection if refractory.

SHOULDER INSTABILITY

Shoulder instability refers to the humeral head moving out of the glenoid fossa secondary to loss of normal function or anatomical stabilisers. It encompasses both frank dislocation and subluxations.

Clinical features:

- Feeling that the joint "pops out"
- Generalised joint pain
- Feeling insecure about shoulder
- Pain on overhead activity
- Posterior instability may complain of recurrent "stingers"

- Assess for features of hypermobility +/− connective tissue disorders

Mechanism of injury:

- Anterior: Blow to abducted, externally rotated and extended arm or microtrauma
- Posterior: Fall onto an outstretched hand (FOOSH), direct contact, seizure
- Other: Atraumatic, related to hypermobility or microtrauma

Examination:

Anterior instability:
- Evidence of laxity – anterior-posterior (AP) draw (glide anterior and posterior).
- Apprehension test + and Relocation test +.
- Beighton score >4/9.
- If traumatic: Initial injury may be associated with other injuries, such as a Bankart lesion, Hill-Sachs lesion, labral injuries and neurological injury. Examination should assess for axillary nerve impairment, rotator cuff tear or a greater tuberosity fracture.
Posterior: Loss of ER
Inferior: Inferior sulcus sign

There are several ways to classify shoulder instability which can aid in guiding further management.

Matsen's classification (3):

- **Traumatic Unilateral** instability associated with a **Bankart** lesion requiring **Surgery** (TUBS)
  - Common after traumatic anterior dislocation
- **Acquired Instability Overuse Syndrome** (AIOS)
  - Secondary to microtrauma from recurrent overhead should activities and may lead to pathology of the labrum
- **Atraumatic Multidirectional** or **Bilateral** instability where **Rehabilitation** is the primary treatment, with an **Inferior** capsular shift performed if surgery is required (AMBRI)
  - Classically seen in patients with hypermobility

The Stanmore triangle recognises three instability patterns (although with some overlap) (4) (Figure 3.2 and Table 3.1).

Investigations:

- X-ray – At least three views (e.g. AP, scapular Y view and axial +/− Stryker notch view) – assess overview of shoulder anatomy and rule out osteoarthritis, assess position of humeral head within glenoid and assess for injuries associated with acute dislocations, e.g. Hill-Sachs lesion or greater tuberosity fracture

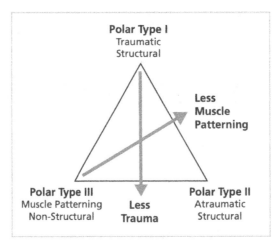

Figure 3.2 Stanmore classification of shoulder instability. (Reproduced with kind permission from *Orthopaedic Trauma, The Stanmore and Royal London Guide*, CRC Press, 2015.)

- Computed tomography (CT) – Mainly indicated after traumatic injury to rule out fractures not visible in X-rays or to assess for bone loss and/or surgical planning
- MRI – Good for soft tissue and labral pathology
- MR arthrogram (MRA) – Most sensitive modality for diagnosing labral tears
- Electromyography (EMG): Can be performed if there is evidence of a peripheral nerve injury and at 6 weeks; if no improvement seen, the patient should be referred to a nerve injury centre.

Management: Traumatic (as per British Elbow and Shoulder Society [BESS] guidelines) (5)

- Closed reduction of the acute dislocation with post-reduction X-rays in two planes and re-evaluation of neurovascular status
- Early mobilisation as pain allows followed by supervised physiotherapy
- In first-time dislocators:
  - Patients aged <25 years should be assessed by an orthopaedic surgeon before 6 weeks with appropriate imaging and risk assessment due to high risk of recurrent dislocations (males under 20 years have 72% chance of recurrent instability)

- Patients aged 25–40 years should be reassessed for instability at 3–6 months
- Patients aged 40–60 years have an increased risk of associated rotator cuff tear so appropriately imaging MRA should be sought
- Arthroscopic repair is as effective as open repair in preventing recurrent dislocation at 2 years

Atraumatic, e.g. AMBRI (6)

- Structured rehabilitation programme with a specialist upper limb physiotherapist focussed on strengthening the dynamic stabilisers of the shoulder +/− taping to reduce extreme ROM
- If symptoms refractory after 6 months of physiotherapy, seek surgical opinion for possible capsular shift.

ADHESIVE CAPSULITIS

"A 60-year-old woman presents to your clinic with a 3-month history of worsening shoulder pain and difficulty sleeping. She is currently taking Ramipril, Metformin and Simvastatin. Please assess."

Adhesive capsulitis is a pathological process characterised by adhesions and contracture of the glenohumeral capsule leading to stiffness, pain and dysfunction. It can be primary (idiopathic) or secondary. Secondary has been associated with trauma, RC disease, cardiovascular disease, diabetes, hypothyroid, metabolic syndrome, female sex and those >40 years.

Phase 1: Painful phase (2–9 months)
Phase 2: Frozen phase with gradual reduction in pain and restriction in ROM (4–12 months)
Phase 3: Thawing phase with improvement in ROM (12–42 months)

Table 3.1 Stanmore classification of shoulder instability and features

Type	Description	Management
Type 1	Traumatic structural	Labral repair
Type 2	Atraumatic structural	Capsular shift
Type 3 (5%)	Muscle patterning, non-structural	Neuromuscular training

There is a considerable overlap in phases, so recent terminology favours the nomenclature "pain predominant" and "stiffness predominant" phases.

Clinical features:

- Insidious onset of general shoulder pain preceding stiffness
- Difficulty sleeping and lying on that shoulder at night
- Pain over deltoid

Examination: Reduced passive ER (early sign), symmetric loss of active and passive ROM

Investigations:

- Fasting lipids, fasting glucose, haemoglobin A1c (HBA1c), thyroid-stimulating hormone (TSH)
- X-ray to rule out osteoarthritis (OA) (main differential diagnosis), avascular necrosis (AVN) or dislocation

Management:

- Education and activity modification
- Analgesia, e.g. Non-steroidal anti-inflammatory drugs (NSAIDs)
- Supervised ROM programme – 6 weeks initially to see if response
  - Stretching
    - Cross-body stretch, pendulum stretch, arm circles
    - Towel stretch for IR
    - Slump stretch forwards onto table
    - ER on door
    - Scapular sets, e.g. scapular clocks
  - Strengthening RC exercises once pain controlled

If symptoms are refractory, discuss further interventions including:

- Corticosteroid injection – May allow reduction of pain to allow further physiotherapy
- Distension, e.g. hydrodilatation
- Arthroscopic capsular release
- Manipulation under anaesthesia

ACROMIOCLAVICULAR JOINT (ACJ) INJURY

Injuries to the ACJ and surrounding structures are common acute injuries of the upper limb.

Mechanism of injury: Fall directly onto acromion, with the arm adducted or FOOSH causing the humerus to be pushed into the acromion.

Clinical features:

- Pain on direct palpation of the ACJ
- Lateral shoulder pain
- Step deformity (due to inferior displacement of humerus)

Examination: Cross-body adduction "scarf" test +, visible step in ACJ if significant displacement, assess horizontal (acromioclavicular ligaments) and vertical (coracoclavicular ligaments) stability

Investigations: X-ray – Bilateral AP and axillary lateral including standing weighted views. Look for:

- Widening of the ACJ >8 mm or >4 mm asymmetry compared with contralateral side
- Increased coracoclavicular distance >13 mm or >5 mm asymmetry
- Superior displacement of the distal clavicle

Grade [Rockwood classification (7)] determines treatment

- Type I: Acromioclavicular (AC) ligament sprain
- Type II: Rupture of AC ligament but coracoclavicular (CC) ligament intact
- Type III: Complete rupture of the AC and CC ligaments
- Type IV: Posterior displacement of clavicle
- Type V: Superior displacement of clavicle and coracoclavicular distance is more than double normal
- Type VI: Inferior displacement of clavicle

Management

- Types I and II – Conservative management with a sling
- Type III – Conservative management with the option of surgery if refractory
- Types IV, V, VI – Refer to surgeons

ΔΔ: Referred pain from cervical or thoracic spine. If chronic, consider distal clavicle osteolysis in weightlifters which presents as an insidious onset of pain with osteopenia on X-ray.

STERNOCLAVICULAR JOINT INJURY

Injuries to the sternoclavicular joint (SCJ) are relatively uncommon injuries to the shoulder girdle, with anterior dislocations being more common than posterior ones.

Mechanism of injury: Fall onto shoulder

Clinical features: Pain and swelling of the sternoclavicular joint. Injuries to the SCJ involve high-energy mechanisms and require thorough assessment for associated injuries, e.g. upper limb neurovascular examination, especially if a posterior dislocation is suspected.

Investigations:

- X-rays: AP and serendipity views (patient is supine, squared and tube tilted at 40° off the vertical)

- CT +/− angiography is now gold standard
- MRI (T2WI) may allow differentiation between SCJ dislocation and physeal injury in younger patients (<25 years)

Management:

- Anterior dislocation:
  - Acute, traumatic and chronic anterior subluxations are usually managed conservatively with ice and sling support for up to 6 weeks. Dislocations and physeal injuries require closed reduction followed by 4 weeks of sling immobilisation
  - Surgery is indicated in those with symptomatic chronic non-reduced anterior dislocations
- Posterior dislocation:
  - Posterior dislocations in the skeletally mature require closed reduction, e.g. abduction traction technique (ideally with thoracic surgery support) followed by 6 weeks of sling immobilisation and then graded rehabilitation. Avoid heavy lifting, elevation or abduction >60° for the first 12 weeks
  - Have a low threshold for surgical referral in possible posterior separation as risk of mediastinal injury to vasculature – e.g. orthopaedic or cardiothoracic referral

Complications: Neurological injuries (brachial plexus, vagus or long thoracic nerve), vascular injuries, thoracic outlet syndrome, respiratory, e.g. pneumothorax or cardiac injuries.

Note: Beware Salter-Harris II fracture in the young as the proximal clavicle epiphysis fuses late.

THORACIC OUTLET SYNDROME

Thoracic outlet syndrome (TOS) describes a group of clinical syndromes causing compression of brachial plexus or subclavian vessels as they pass through the thoracic outlet.

Clinical features: Majority are neurogenic (non-radicular pain and upper limb weakness and/or paraesthesia). Other symptoms reported include venous (engorgement or swelling in arm) and arterial (cool, pale hand) phenomena.

Aetiology:

- The majority are secondary to soft tissue abnormalities, e.g. scalene muscle abnormality
- Osseous, e.g. cervical rib
- Vascular, e.g. aneurysm
- Don't miss: Pancoast tumour (look for Horner's syndrome), Paget-Schroetter (upper arm deep vein thrombosis (DVT) in the axillary or subclavian vein secondary to abnormal costoclavicular ligament)

The thoracic outlet is comprised of three distinct spaces which can be potentially affected (Figure 3.3).

1. Interscalene – Affects brachial plexus and subclavian artery

Thoracic outlet syndrome

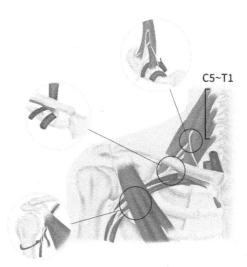

C5~T1

Figure 3.3 The three distinct spaces in thoracic outlet syndrome comprise the interscalene space (*top circle*), the costoclavicular space (*middle circle*) and retropectoralis (*bottom circle*).

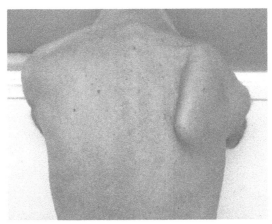

Figure 3.4 Patient with right scapula winging evidenced by the accentuated medial border of the scapula. (This figure was published in *A Comprehensive Guide to Sports Physiology and Injury Management*, Porter and Wilson, page 296, Copyright Elsevier, 2021.)

2. Costoclavicular – Brachial plexus, subclavian artery and vein
3. Retropectoralis minor – Brachial plexus and axillary artery and vein

Examination: Assess skin, muscle atrophy, supraclavicular palpation, Adson's test (interscalene), Wright test (retropectoralis major) and Roos test (all aetiologies), Auscultate chest (Pancoast).

Note: Tends to impact C8 and T1 (90% cases), therefore, assess for ulnar nerve involvement (sensory and motor) or median nerve involvement (motor involvement but spares sensory which is innervated by C5,6,7).

Investigations:

- Chest X-ray (CXR) and C spine X-ray – assess for presence of a cervical rib, C7 transverse (TV) process, Pancoast tumour at apex
- Vascular – US or CT angiography (CTA)/MRA
- MRI – soft tissue abnormalities
- EMG and nerve conduction studies (NCS)

Management largely depends on the aetiology of the condition:

- Activity modification, analgesia, rehabilitation and mobilisation exercises
- Consider surgical referral depending on aetiology and for those refractory to conservative management

ΔΔ: T1 root pathology, peripheral nerve entrapment

SCAPULAR WINGING

Scapular winging results due to a dysfunction in the stabilising muscles of the scapula causing an abnormal scapular motion.

Medial scapular winging is the most common – Secondary to long thoracic nerve injury causing a weak serratus anterior which leads to weak scapular protraction, e.g. brachial neuritis.

Lateral scapular winging is secondary to an injury to the spinal accessory (XI) nerve causing trapezius dysfunction, therefore, a weak superior and mediating force. It is commonly iatrogenic, e.g. after neck surgery, therefore it is important to look for scars of previous surgery.

Clinical features: Shoulder pain, weakness, neuropathic pain if brachial neuritis.

You can accentuate winging by asking patient to perform a push-up against a wall (Figure 3.4).

Investigations:

- EMG
- X-rays to rule out structural abnormalities

Management:

- Most isolated serratus anterior palsies respond well to conservative management of ROM and strengthening exercises.
- Trapezius palsy may require surgical referral for exploration and/or nerve repair.

ΔΔ: Peripheral nerve entrapment, cervical spine disease, familial scapulohumeral dystrophy (bilateral)

REFERENCES

1. Snyder SJ, Karzel RP, Del Pizzo W, Ferkel RD, Friedman MJ. SLAP lesions of the shoulder. *Arthroscopy*. 1990;6:274–9.
2. Ellman H. Diagnosis and treatment of incomplete rotator cuff tears. *Clin Orthop Relat Res*. 1990(254): 64–74.
3. Matsen FA 3rd, Harryman DT 2nd, Sidles JA. Mechanics of glenohumeral instability. *Clin. Sports Med*. 1991;10(4): 783–8.

4. Lewis A, Kitamura T, Bailey JIL. The classification of shoulder instability: New light through old windows! *Curr Orthop*. 2004;18:97–108.

5. Brownson P, Donaldson O, Fox M, Rees JL, Rangan A, Jaggi A, et al. BESS/BOA patient care pathways: traumatic anterior shoulder instability. *Shoulder Elbow*. 2015;7(3):214–26.

6. Noorani A, Goldring M, Jaggi A, Gibson J, Rees J, Bateman M, et al. BESS/BOA patient care pathways: atraumatic shoulder instability. *Shoulder Elbow*. 2019; 11(1):60–70.

7. Rockwood C. Fractures and dislocations of the shoulder. In: *Fractures in Adults*. Philadelphia: Lippincott; 1984: pp. 860–910.

The main differential diagnoses for elbow pain are summarised in Table 4.1.

TENDINOPATHY OF COMMON EXTENSOR ORIGIN

Overuse injury at the origin of the common extensor tendon at the lateral epicondyle of the elbow. Commonly involvement is of extensor carpi radialis brevis (ECRB) (can also be extensor digitorum [ED] or extensor carpi ulnaris [ECU]).

Clinical features: insidious onset of pain on and proximal to the lateral epicondyle after unaccustomed or eccentric activity involving wrist extension and gripping

Examination:

- Localised tenderness over the common extensor origin
- Pain on repeated wrist extension or resisted wrist extension
- Pain on resisted middle finger extension

Investigations: US = hypoechoic change in the tendon, thickened tendon, neovascularisation

Management:

- Patient education: 80% resolve by 12 months
- Activity modification and analgesia
- Progressive strengthening programme of forearm extensor muscles
- Bracing can be considered if relieves symptoms
- Technique or training load adjustment

Reserve further investigations or second-line treatments (e.g. extra corporeal shock wave [ECSW] or autologous blood injection [ABI]) for refractory cases.

ΔΔ:

- C-spine radiculopathy at C6–7
- Radial tunnel syndrome (compression of the posterior interosseous nerve [PIN] at the lateral intermuscular septum characterised by **pain** only and no motor dysfunction. Pain is more distal then CEO tendinopathy and EMG is normal as fibres are unmyelinated). Note supinator syndrome is PIN compression at the arcade of Frohse

OSTEOCHONDRITIS DISSECANS OF THE CAPITELLUM

This is an injury secondary to repetitive microtrauma of immature capitellum causing separation of articular cartilage and subchondral bone. It is common in adolescent gymnasts and throwing

Mechanism of injury: repetitive compression injury

Clinical features:

- Insidious onset of lateral elbow pain related to activity
- Mechanical symptoms, e.g. clicking or locking
- Loss of extension

Examination:

- Loss of extension
- Tender to palpation just above radial head +/− effusion

Investigations:

- X-ray: Findings may be occult initially. Findings may include flattening or indistinct lucency around the contour surface. More advanced changes include fragmentation and density changes (see Chapter 18)
- MRI is the modality of choice with a high intensity rim at the interface between the fragment and the bone on T2WI or a focal osteochondral defect filled with fluid if detached

Clanton classification (1):

Type I   – Depressed osteochondral fracture
Type II   – Fragment attached by osseous bridge
Type III – Detached non-displaced fragment
Type IV   – Displaced fragment

Management: Depends on grade

- Conservative management for stable lesions:
  - Cease provoking activity, analgesia, graded return to activities with loading activities last

DOI: 10.1201/9781003163701-6

Table 4.1 Differential diagnoses of elbow and forearm pain according to location

Lateral elbow	Medial elbow	Posterior elbow
• Common extensor origin (CEO) tendinopathy • Osteochondritis dissecans (radiocapitellar joint) • Lateral collateral ligament injury • Radial head OA • Radial tunnel or PIN syndrome • Referred pain – C6/C7	• Common flexor origin (Clinical features) tendinopathy • Medial epicondyle apophysitis, bone stress injury • Valgus stress causing ulnar collateral ligament injury • Snapping ulnar nerve or triceps • Ulnar nerve • Referred pain – C8, T1	• Olecranon bursitis • Triceps tendinopathy • Posterior impingement • Gouty tophus

OA, osteoarthritis; PIN, posterior interosseous nerve.

- Surgical referral for microfracture if unstable lesions or refractory cases

TENDINOPATHY OF COMMON FLEXOR ORIGIN

Overuse injury of the flexor-pronator muscle group at the origin of the common extensor tendon at the medial epicondyle of the elbow. The flexor-pronator mass consists of pronator teres, flexor carpi radialis (FCR), flexor digitorum superficialis (FDS), palmaris longus and flexor carpi ulnaris (FCU).

Clinical features:

- Activity-related (especially throwing) medial elbow pain of gradual onset
- Weakness of grip strength
- +/– paraesthesia in the ulnar nerve distribution

Examination:

- Pain to palpation just distal and anterior to the medical epicondyle over the insertion of the flexor-pronator muscles
- Pain provocation on resisted wrist flexion and pronation
- Reduced grip strength
- Include cervical spine assessment in examination

Investigations:

- Diagnosis is usually clinical
- US or MRI useful to delineate soft tissue structures. US may show hypoechoic change in the tendon, thickened tendon, neovascularisation

Management:

- Patient education
- Activity modification and analgesia
- Progressive strengthening programme forearm flexor muscles
- Technique or training load adjustment

ΔΔ: Ulnar nerve pathology, ulnar collateral ligament instability, C-spine radiculopathy at T1

VALGUS EXTENSION OVERLOAD SYNDROME

Clinical syndrome typically seen in adolescent throwing athletes involving injury to the ulnar collateral ligament (Figure 4.1) +/– radiocapitellar or ulnohumeral joint. Valgus extension overload syndrome can subsequently → osteochondritis dissecans of radiocapitellar joint. This can cause restriction of full extension.

Clinical features:

- Medial/posterior elbow pain on throwing
- Pain on full extension
- Restriction of movement of full extension

Examination:

- Localised tenderness over posteromedial elbow joint
- Pain provocation with valgus stress when elbow is extended and at 30° of flexion
- Crepitus
- Loss of full extension

Investigations:

- X-rays: If chronic assess for osteophytes, osteochondral defects of the capitellum or ossification of the UCL
- MRI is normally the investigation of choice. Partial or complete of the UCL can be demonstrated by ligament discontinuity, increased signal intensity of the fibres and surrounding oedema. Osteochondral fragments can also be assessed of the radiocapitellar joint

Management:

- Relative rest from provocative manoeuvres and throwing and analgesia
- Technique modification
- Flexor pronator strengthening programme

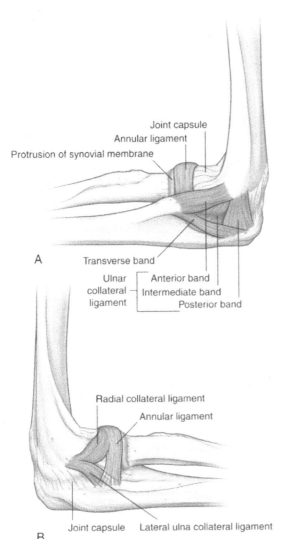

A

- Joint capsule
- Annular ligament
- Protrusion of synovial membrane
- Transverse band
- Ulnar collateral ligament
  - Anterior band
  - Intermediate band
  - Posterior band

B

- Radial collateral ligament
- Annular ligament
- Joint capsule
- Lateral ulna collateral ligament

Figure 4.1 Medial (A) and lateral (B) aspects of the left elbow showing the joint capsule and the radial and ulnar collateral ligaments. (This figure was published in a *Comprehensive Guide to Sports Physiology and Injury Management*, Porter and Wilson, page 305, Copyright Elsevier, 2021.)

- Surgery if full thickness tear or refractory symptoms

DISTAL BICEPS TENDON TEAR

The distal biceps tendon attaches to the radial tuberosity of the elbow (the short head inserts distally and the long head attaches proximally).

Mechanisms of acute injury include forced extension of the elbow with the arm in supination or elbow extension during heavy lifting.

Clinical features:

- Sudden pain over the antecubital fossa with loss of function of elbow flexion
- Ecchymosis
- Visible contracted biceps muscle belly 'reverse Popeye sign'
- On examination there may be a palpable gap in the antecubital fossa and there will be pain and weakness on resisted elbow flexion and supination
- Hook test can be used to locate the lateral edge of the biceps tendon and you should be able to insert your finger around this landmark if intact

Investigations:

- X-rays: AP and lateral can be helpful to rule out alternative pathology, e.g. acute fracture or to identify an avulsion
- US and MRI can identify a partial or complete rupture or to assess for features of chronic tendinopathy

Management:

- In young patients, these injuries require early surgical intervention within 2 weeks to reattach the tendon to the radial tuberosity, followed by a progressive rehabilitation programme

REFERENCE

1. Clanton TO, DeLee JC. Osteochondritis dissecans. History, pathophysiology and current treatment concepts. *Clin Orthop Relat Res.* 1982(167):50–64.

The main differential diagnoses of wrist pain are summarised in Table 5.1.

RADIAL-SIDED PATHOLOGY

SCAPHOID FRACTURE

"A 23-year-old has fallen onto their outstretched right hand during a night out. They present to A&E minors with pain and reduced movement of their wrist. Please assess."

The scaphoid is the most commonly fractured carpal bone. The scaphoid receives its blood supply from the dorsal carpal branch of the radial artery distally, therefore proximal pole fractures have a high risk of non-union (Figure 5.1).

Mechanism of injury: Commonly FOOSH

Clinical features: Pain of the dorsal wrist, swelling and loss of grip strength

Examination:

1. Anatomical snuffbox tenderness
2. Pain on axial load (telescoping)
3. Tenderness of scaphoid tubercle

Also, pain with resisted pronation

Investigations:

1. X-rays are first line: Dedicated scaphoid views including posteroanterior (PA), oblique, lateral and posteroanterior view angled (Zitters) – assess for fracture line and displacement. May initially be negative so repeat in 7–10 days
2. Magnetic resonance imaging (MRI) – secondary investigation if initial X-rays negative
3. Computed tomography (CT) – second-line modality which can exclude a fracture

Classification:

1. Herbert classification (1)
   - A: Acute, stable
   - B: Acute, unstable
   - C: Delayed union
   - D: Established non-union
2. Mayo classification (2)
   - Middle (70%), distal (20%) and proximal (10%)
3. Russe classification (3)
   - Type I: Horizontal oblique fracture (distal, middle, proximal)
   - Type II: Transverse fracture
   - Type III: Vertical oblique fracture

Management:

1. Unstable and non-displaced:
   - Immobilise in a scaphoid plaster and high arm sling and refer to fracture clinic for orthopaedic review. A scaphoid plaster extends from the angle of the elbow to the metacarpal heads and around the base of the thumb to below the interphalangeal joint
   - Immobilise for:
     - 3 months if injury to the distal pole
     - 4 months if injury is to the waist (most common)
     - 5 months if injury is to the proximal pole
2. Unstable or proximal pole: operative fixation using percutaneous screw or ORIF (high risk of avascular necrosis [AVN] or non-union)
3. Rehabilitation thereafter to improve stiffness and strength deficits

Complications: AVN, non-union, osteoarthritis

DE QUERVAIN'S TENOSYNOVITIS

"A 34-year-old woman who is 4 months post-partum presents with unilateral wrist pain, making it difficult to pick up and feed her baby. There are no neurological symptoms, and she complains of some swelling on the dorsum of her hand."

De Quervain's tenosynovitis is a stenosing tenosynovitis of the 1st dorsal compartment containing extensor pollicis brevis (EPB) and abductor

DOI: 10.1201/9781003163701-7

Table 5.1 Differential diagnoses of hand and wrist pathology according to location

Radial		Ulnar	
Dorsal	**Volar**	**Dorsal**	**Volar**
• 1st CMC OA • Scaphoid fracture • De Quervain's tenosynovitis • Intersection syndrome	• Scaphoid fracture	• TFCC tear • Scapholunate dissociation • ECU subluxation	• Ulnar nerve compression in Guyon's canal • Hook of hamate fracture

CMC, carpometacarpal; OA, osteoarthritis; TFCC, triangular fibrocartilage complex; ECU, extensor carpi ulnaris.

pollicis longus (APL) at the level of the radial styloid (Figure 5.2). Extensor retinaculum swelling causes tendon friction.

Mechanism of injury: Common after overuse, e.g. racquet sports or postpartum

Clinical features: swelling, tenderness on the radial side of the wrist (Figure 5.3), pain on thumb and wrist movement

Examination: Palpable crepitus, Finkelstein test +

Investigations: Not normally required, but ultrasound (US) can demonstrate oedema and thickening of APL and EPB at the radial styloid or increased fluid within the tendon sheath of the first extensor compartment

X-rays can help to rule out differentials, e.g. 1st carpometacarpal osteoarthritis

Management:

1. Education
2. Activity modification – avoid aggravating activity
3. Non-steroidal anti-inflammatories (NSAIDs)
4. Thumb spica
5. Strengthening exercises
6. Corticosteroid injection
7. Refractory: Surgical referral for consideration of release

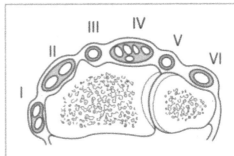

I Abductor pollicis longus and extensor pollicis brevis
II Extensor carpi radialis longus and brevis
III Extensor pollicis longus
IV Extensor digitorum communis and extensor indicis
V Extensor digiti minimi
VI Extensor carpi ulnaris

Figure 5.2 The six dorsal compartments of the hand and their respective contents. (Reproduced with kind permission from *Orthopaedic Trauma: The Stanmore and Royal London Guide*, CRC Press, 2015.)

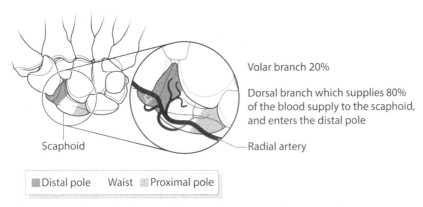

Volar branch 20%

Dorsal branch which supplies 80% of the blood supply to the scaphoid, and enters the distal pole

Scaphoid

Radial artery

■ Distal pole   Waist   ■ Proximal pole

Figure 5.1 Scaphoid fracture location and blood supply.

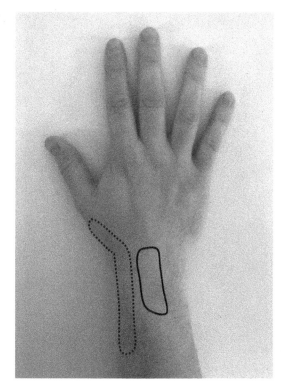

Figure 5.3 Location of pain in De Quervain's tenosynovitis (*dotted line*) versus intersection syndrome (*solid line*).

INTERSECTION SYNDROME

Intersection syndrome is an inflammatory tenosynovitis between the 1st dorsal compartment (EPB and APL) and the 2nd dorsal compartment (extensor carpi radialis brevis [ECRB] and extensor carpi radialis longus [ECRL]) of the hand. It is common after repetitive wrist flexion, e.g. the classical description is in rower's 'oarsmen's wrist' approximately 6–8 cm from Lister's tubercle (Figure 5.3). It is less common than De Quervain's tenosynovitis.

Clinical features: Pain, crepitus and swelling over the dorsum of the wrist

Examination:

- Pain with resisted wrist extension and thumb extension
- Crepitus and tenderness on dorsoradial forearm
- Often Finklestein's test will be + as well

Investigations: If refractory or unclear diagnosis

Management:

1. Activity modification
2. NSAIDs
3. Wrist splint – neutral position
4. Change technique or load, e.g. smaller oar handle, thumb position on top

5. Corticosteroid injection
6. Refractory: Imaging +/– surgical referral

CARPAL TUNNEL SYNDROME

Carpal tunnel syndrome (CTS) is a compression neuropathy of the median nerve within the carpal tunnel of the wrist.

The carpal tunnel consists of: the median nerve, eight flexor tendons (flexor digitorum profundus [FDP] and flexor digitorum superficialis [FDS]) and flexor pollicis longus (FPL).

Risk factors: Type II diabetes mellitus (T2DM), hypothyroidism, rheumatoid arthritis, pregnancy, acromegaly, chronic renal failure, alcohol, female, age

- *Ask about these in the history including symptoms of hypothyroidism, alcohol intake, possible pregnancy*

Clinical features:

- Pain and/or paraesthesia in radial 3.5 digits, which can radiate to the forearm
- Nocturnal symptoms
- Difficulty gripping

Examination:

- Assess thenar eminence bulk – wasted if longstanding
- Weak opposition of thumb and little finger
- Weak thumb abduction
- Reduced sensation top of index finger
- Special tests: Phalen's test, Tinel's test, Durkan's test +

Investigations: it is normally a clinical diagnosis. NCS/EMG can help to confirm

Investigations of potential risk factors: consider doing bloods, such as a blood sugar (BM), fasting glucose, thyroid function tests (TFTs), urea and electrolytes (U&E) and beta HCG (pregnancy test)

Management:

1. Activity modification
2. Treat cause or education regarding cause, e.g. likely to improve after postpartum period
3. Analgesia
4. Night splints (wrist in neutral)
5. Occupational therapy or hand physiotherapy referral if interfering with work or activities of daily living (ADLs)

If refractory to above consider:

6. Steroid + local anaesthetic (LA) injection (see Chapter 13)
7. Surgical referral if refractory to consider decompression

ΔΔ: Neurological disease, e.g. multiple sclerosis (MS), active inflammatory joint disease, peripheral limb ischaemia, e.g. thoracic outlet syndrome (TOS), cervical nerve root entrapment.

ULNAR-SIDED PATHOLOGY

TRIANGULAR FIBROCARTILAGE COMPLEX (TFCC) TEARS

The TFCC is a load-bearing structure between the lunate, triquetrum and ulnar head. It acts as a stabiliser for the ulnar aspect of wrist.

TFCC injury is commonly secondary to traction of the ulnar wrist but it can also be traumatic. It is associated with a positive ulnar variance, which refers to when the ulnar projects more distally relative to the radius (see the box and Figure 5.4).

Ulnar variance

The styloid process of the radius is normally more distal than that of the ulnar, but with the forearm supinated they are approximately at the same level. This relationship is known as ulnar variance and can be altered secondary to growth abnormalities or injury.

Clinical features:

- Ulnar wrist pain especially on compressive loading, +/− clicking
- Instability
- Weak grip

Examination:

- Swelling of ulnar wrist
- Special tests: Compression test (wrist dorsiflexion and ulnar deviation) +, ulnar fovea sign +, press test +, ulnomeniscal triquetral dorsal glide test, piano key test + if unstable

Investigations:

- X-ray to assess ulnar variance, any volar tilt of scaphoid and lunate (lunotriquetral ligament torn) and rule out differentials, e.g. ulnar styloid fracture
- MRI +/− arthrogram
- Arthroscopy is gold standard as MRI may miss small tears

Classification: Palmer classification (4) – Class 1 are traumatic and Class 2 are degenerative

Management:

1. Immobilisation with brace 3–6 weeks
2. Analgesia
3. Strengthening exercises – wrist flexion and extension
4. Surgical referral if unstable or refractory to conservative management by 6 months
   - Options include arthroscopic repair, debridement, ulnar shortening, Wafer procedure

ΔΔ: Ulnar styloid fractures, ulnar impaction syndrome (commonly bone signal change in ulnar side of proximal lunate or triquetrum), distal radioulnar joint chrondral lesions or osteoarthritis, Kienböck disease.

EXTENSOR CARPI ULNARIS (ECU) TENDON SUBLUXATION

The ECU is part of the 6th dorsal compartment of the hand and stabilises the distal radial-ulnar joint. Injury is secondary to overuse causing the ECU to sublux from its subsheath.

Clinical features: Pain and/or 'snapping' of the ulnar wrist

Examination:

- Visible or palpable subluxation on wrist supination, which reduces with pronation (cobra test)

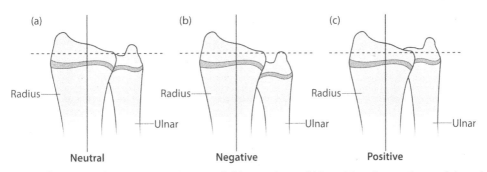

Figure 5.4 Illustration demonstrating (a) neutral, (b) negative and (c) positive ulnar variance of the wrist.

- Synergy test + for pain (patient radially deviates their thumb against resistance)

Investigations:

- US can be used to dynamically assess instability and snapping in real-time
- MRI may demonstrate tendonitis or tears of the ECU

Management:

1. Wrist splint (pronation and radial deviation) for 4 weeks following by a progressive strengthening programme
2. Surgical referral if refractory symptoms or a torn sheath

ΔΔ: TFCC tear

ULNAR NERVE COMPRESSION AT GUYON'S CANAL

Compressive neuropathy of the ulnar nerve at Guyon's canal in the wrist (Figure 5.5).

Common in cyclists 'handlebar palsy' and repeated catching sports.

Also be aware of possible underlying aetiology, such as a ganglion cyst, hook of hamate fracture or ulnar artery thrombosis.

Zone 1	Mixed motor and sensory	Ganglia, hook of hamate fracture
Zone 2	Motor	Ganglia, hook of hamate fracture
Zone 3	Sensory	Ulnar artery thrombosis

Clinical features:

- Pain and paraesthesia in little finger and ulnar half of ring finger
- Weak intrinsics, e.g. crossing fingers
- Motor and sensory involvement depends on which zone is affected (see box)

Examination:

- Clawed ring and little finger
- Intrinsic weakness – weak pinch, Froment's sign +, Wartenberg sign +
- Palpate hamate for pain suggesting a fracture
- Allen test to assess for ulnar artery thrombosis

Investigations:

- X-ray (hamate fracture)
- CT (hamate fracture)
- MRI (ganglion cyst)
- US or MRA (thrombosis)

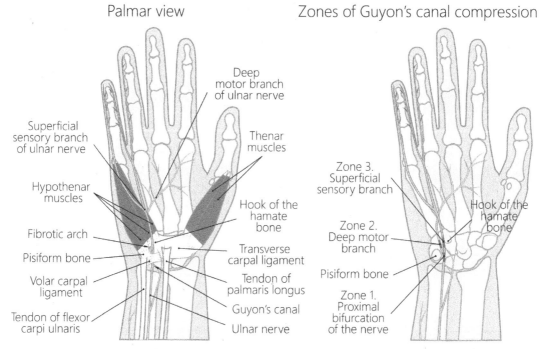

GUYON'S CANAL SYNDROME
(ENTRAPMENT OF THE ULNAR NERVE)

Palmar view

Zones of Guyon's canal compression

Superficial sensory branch of ulnar nerve

Hypothenar muscles

Fibrotic arch

Pisiform bone

Volar carpal ligament

Tendon of flexor carpi ulnaris

Deep motor branch of ulnar nerve

Thenar muscles

Hook of the hamate bone

Transverse carpal ligament

Tendon of palmaris longus

Guyon's canal

Ulnar nerve

Zone 3. Superficial sensory branch

Zone 2. Deep motor branch

Pisiform bone

Zone 1. Proximal bifurcation of the nerve

Hook of the hamate bone

Figure 5.5 Guyon's canal syndrome. Anatomy surrounding Guyon's canal and the different zones of entrapment. (Shutterstock ID 499824424.)

Electromyography (EMG)/nerve conduction studies (NCS)– can help confirm diagnosis

Management:

1. Activity modification and change handlebar grip and bike set up
2. NSAIDs
3. Splinting
4. Surgical referral if refractory for decompression

FINGER CLINICAL CASES

A representation of some of the digital tendinous structures is shown in Figure 5.6.

Mallet finger

- Injury to extensor insertion at the distal interphalangeal (DIP) joint, e.g. ball striking end of finger
- Either bony avulsion or tendon tear
- Clinical features: inability to extend DIP joint
- Management: splint in neutral (bony) or extension (tendon)

Jersey finger

- Injury to long flexor insertion at the DIP joint of flexor digitorum profundus
- Finger held in extension relative to others
- Clinical features: Inability to flex DIP
- Investigations: X-ray to exclude avulsion
- Management: Surgical referral

Trigger finger

- Stenosing tenosynovitis in flexor tendon impacting A1 pulley
- Ass: T2DM, amyloidosis, hypothyroidism
- Clinical features: painful clicking and locking of fingers during flexion, there may be a nodule present

- It is a clinical diagnosis but US can help confirm
- Management: Conservative management – including splinting, corticosteroid injection +/− surgical referral if refractory

Disruption of central slip

- Disruption of the central slip of extensor digitorum communis tendon causes the lateral bands to migrate volarly
- Examination:
  - Elson test assesses central slip integrity if rupture is suspected. Fix the proximal interphalangeal (PIP) joint at 90° and ask the patient to extend the DIP joint. If the central slip is injured, then there is fixed extension of the DIP and it feels rigid due to increased unopposed pull of the lateral bands
- Management:
  - If <4 weeks then trial conservative management by splinting the PIP in extension for 3–6 weeks and referral to a hand surgeon. After splinting assess for an extensor lag
- Complications of a missed injury can lead to a Bountonnière deformity

Stener lesion

- Thumb metacarpophalangeal joint (MCP) dislocations can be associated with ulnar collateral ligament injury or an avulsion fracture, also known as 'game-keeper's' thumb
- A Stener lesion occurs when the distal stump comes to lie above the adductor aponeurosis which results in chronic instability in adduction (Figure 5.7)
- Clinical features include pain located on the ulnar aspect of the MCP joint and pain on pinch or a weak pinch grip

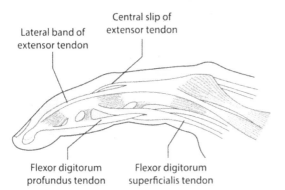

Central slip of extensor tendon

Lateral band of extensor tendon

Flexor digitorum profundus tendon

Flexor digitorum superficialis tendon

Figure 5.6 The relationship of the digital tendinous structures. (Reproduced with kind permission from *Orthopaedic Trauma: The Stanmore and Royal London Guide*, CRC Press, 2015.)

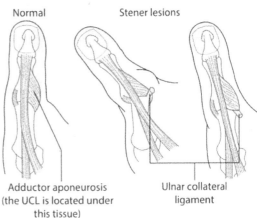

Normal   Stener lesions

Adductor aponeurosis (the UCL is located under this tissue)

Ulnar collateral ligament

Figure 5.7 Ulnar collateral ligament injury mechanism and formation of a Stener lesion. (Reproduced with kind permission from *Orthopaedic Trauma: The Stanmore and Royal London Guide*, CRC Press, 2015.)

- Investigations: X-rays (PA, lateral and oblique) to assess for an avulsion, US and MRI can be helpful if findings in doubt
- All Stener lesions require operative repair

REFERENCES

1. Herbert TJ, Fisher WE. Management of the fractured scaphoid using a new bone screw. *J Bone Joint Surg Br.* 1984;66(1):114–23.
2. Cooney WP, Dobyns JH, Linscheid RL. Fractures of the scaphoid: A rational approach to management. *Clin Orthop Relat Res.* 1980;(149):90–7.
3. Russe O. Fracture of the carpal navicular. Diagnosis, non-operative treatment, and operative treatment. *J Bone Joint Surg Am.* 1960;42-A:759–68.
4. Palmer AK. Triangular fibrocartilage complex lesions: A classification. *J Hand Surg Am.* 1989;14:594–606.

CERVICAL SPINE

CERVICAL RADICULOPATHY

"A 52-year-old painter and decorator has been referred by his General Practitioner (GP) with persistent aching in his right arm with some occasional pins and needles and numbness. He is now finding it difficult to work as his arm feels weaker than normal."

Cervical spine nerve root compression is commonly caused by degenerative cervical spondylosis or a disc herniation. C7 is most common.

Clinical features:

- Neck pain of insidious onset
- Unilateral shoulder or arm pain (non-dermatomal)
- Unilateral paraesthesia and/or weakness

Examination:

- Restricted cervical spine movements
- Neurological signs in keeping with nerve root affected (see Table 6.1)

See Figure 2.3 for upper limb dermatomes.

- Spurling test + (ask the patient to systematically move their neck into extension and then lateral flexion and then place axial compression on the head)
- Assess for Horner's syndrome and Pancoast tumour if T1 involvement
- Upper limb tension tests may be +
- Ensure no signs of myelopathy including clumsiness, ataxia, upper motor neuron (UMN) signs (Babinski +, Hoffman's sign +, hyperreflexia)

Investigations:

1. X-rays: Cervical spine anteroposterior (AP), lateral and oblique (osteophytes, canal stenosis), Chest X-ray (CXR) to assess for a Pancoast tumour
2. Magnetic resonance imaging (MRI): assess for disc herniation or nerve root compression
3. Electromyography (EMG)/nerve conduction studies (NCS) if you suspect a peripheral nerve lesion as an alternative diagnosis

Management:

1. Education – majority improve without surgical intervention
2. Relative rest and activity modification
3. Analgesia – non-steroidal anti-inflammatories (NSAIDs)
4. Physiotherapy referral for possible mobilisation exercises
5. Occupational therapy (OT) referral if symptoms are affecting work
6. If refractory, consider nerve root block or surgical referral

ΔΔ: Peripheral nerve entrapment, shingles, Parsonage-Turner syndrome, thoracic outlet syndrome (TOS)

CENTRAL CORD SYNDROME

This is a type of incomplete cord injury syndrome, typically secondary to trauma, and is also more common in those with underlying cervical spondylosis.

Clinical features:

- Initial flaccid weakness, which is followed by:
- Lower motor neuron (LMN) paralysis of the upper limbs (damage to anterior horn cells) with
- UMN (spastic) paralysis of the lower limbs (due to interruption of descending corticospinal tracts) and
- Intact perianal sensation (sacral sparing) +/− bladder control

Investigations:

- X-ray and computed tomography (CT) may show cervical spondylosis or an acute fracture

DOI: 10.1201/9781003163701-8

Table 6.1 Clinical features of cervical spine nerve root entrapment

	C4	C5	C6	C7	C8	T1
Sensory	Cape distribution	Regimental badge	Thumb	Middle finger	Little finger	Ulnar forearm
Pain	Lower neck, trapezius	Lateral arm	Dorsolateral arm	Forearm, middle finger	Little finger and medial forearm	Ulnar forearm
Motor	–	Deltoid, elbow flexion	Elbow flexion, wrist extension	Triceps	Finger flexion	Finger adduction
Reflexes	–	Biceps	Brachioradialis	Triceps	–	–
Other						+/– Horner's

- MRI will show increased signal in the cord at the level affected on T2 weighted-imaging (T2WI), and may also demonstrate an associated cord haematoma or haemorrhagic contusions (see Chapter 18)

Management of acute traumatic central cord syndrome depends on the presence of mechanical instability or ongoing cord compression where surgical intervention is required.

CERVICAL MYELOPATHY

"A 72-year-old woman is referred because of an insidious onset of difficulty gripping objects with her right hand. She is now struggling to do up shirt buttons or tie her shoelaces. The GP initially suspected carpal tunnel syndrome, but on close questioning she also admits her walking is becoming more unsteady."

Cervical myelopathy is due to compression of the spinal cord (or diminished vascular supply) commonly secondary to degenerative cervical spondylosis. Other causes include malignancy, spinal abscess and cervical kyphosis.

Clinical features: (Normally requires 30% compression to cause symptoms)

- Neck pain
- Weakness and reduced manual dexterity/clumsiness
- Paraesthesia
- Unsteady gait
- Urinary retention (late sign)

Note: Upper extremity signs are often unilateral, whilst lower extremity signs are commonly bilateral. Cervical myelopathy can also present with a radiculopathy as well.

Examination:

- Gait: Romberg's test +, difficulty with heel-to-toe walking, may have spasticity or a broad-based gait

- 'Myelopathy hand' which is loss of adduction and extension of the ulnar two or three digits – test with the finger escape sign
- Sensory: Disturbances may include reduced pain or altered temperature (spinothalamic), proprioception or vibration (dorsal columns) but preserved light touch
- Motor: Reduced dexterity in hands, e.g. grip and release test. Flaccid weakness at the level of the lesion and spastic weakness below the lesion
- UMN signs: Hyperreflexia, Hoffman's test +, Clonus, Babinski +

Investigations:

- X-rays: Cervical spine AP, lateral and oblique views (look for osteophytes, canal stenosis: Pavlov ratio < 0.8)
- MRI: Spinal cord high signal on T2WI

Management: Depends on the grade (Nurick classification)

Conservative management is acceptable in mild cases with no functional impairment:

- Education
- Activity modification
- NSAIDs, e.g. naproxen

Surgical referral for ongoing monitoring and consideration of decompression in those with severe functional impairment and those with disease at level C1–2.

ΔΔ: Spinal tumour, motor neuron disease, multiple sclerosis, syringomyelia, cerebellar syndrome, vitamin B12 deficiency, diabetic neuropathy.

THORACIC SPINE AND CHEST

RIB STRESS FRACTURE

"A rower comes to see you complaining of right sided 'chest pain' during training and competition. He denies shortness of breath or palpitations. He says

the pain can be aggravated by breathing, twisting and doing upper body exercises in the gym. He has pinpoint tenderness over his 6th rib."

Stress fractures of the rib are commonly located at the anterolateral portion of 4th–8th ribs.

They can arise after a period of increased load (frequency, volume or intensity of training), suboptimal technique or due to reduced thoracic range of movement (ROM).

Clinical features:

- Pain in the front, side or back of the chest wall
- Pain on deep inspiration, coughing or rolling over

Examination:

- Pinpoint tenderness over the affected area, rib spring +
- Ensure you also perform a cardiorespiratory examination and assess for evidence of a deep vein thrombosis (DVT)

Investigations: As per bone stress investigations – bloods including full blood count (FBC), urea and electrolytes (U&E), liver function tests (LFTs), bone profile, vitamin D and thyroid function tests (TFTs).

Imaging: X-rays are insensitive to early bone stress lesions <6 weeks. If short-duration symptoms (<6 weeks) then use MRI: Bone marrow oedema on T2WI or short-tau inversion recovery (STIR)

Management:

- Education and relative rest
- Analgesia
- Correct any calcium or vitamin D deficiency
- Continue cardiovascular (CV) training to maintain fitness, e.g. cycling
- Technique analysis including correction of any biomechanical errors such as high pull or over-reaching
- Strengthening programme focussing on serratus anterior (antagonist to external oblique), e.g. pull down exercises

ΔΔ: Cardiac causes, gastro-oesophageal reflux disease, pulmonary embolus, shingles, Scheuermann's disease, costochondritis

LUMBAR SPINE

Differential diagnoses of pain in the lumbar spine are shown in Table 6.2.

SPONDYLOLYSIS/BONE STRESS OF THE PARS INTERARTICULARIS

"A 15-year-old gymnast presents with lower back pain following a recent training camp which came on gradually over a few days. Their pain is worse on landing from apparatus and any twisting movements and it persists for a day or two after. She reports no neurological symptoms."

"A 17-year-old fast bowler presents with unilateral back stiffness and pain when bowling 3 weeks after a recent training camp. Please assess."

Spondylolysis is a defect in the pars interarticularis of the neural arch. It is common in sports with repeated hyperextension, e.g. cricket bowling or gymnastics and it correlates with periods of increased spinal load at a time of bony immaturity. Injury of the pars interarticularis can occur on a spectrum of severity from active bone stress to a chronic defect including non-united stress fractures.

Clinical features: Unilateral (sometimes bilateral) lower back pain on spinal extension, worsened by activity and relieved by rest.

Examination:

- Stork test +
- Quadrant test +
- Tenderness to palpation over area
- May have lordotic posture with tight hamstrings

Investigations:

1. Workup for bone stress including FBC, U&E, bone profile, vitamin D, TFTs (although many are load related)
2. Imaging
   a. X-rays are insensitive to early bone stress lesions <6 weeks. Chronic defects can be seen on oblique X-rays as the 'Scotty dog sign'

Table 6.2 Differential diagnoses for lumbar spine pain		
Common	**Uncommon**	**Do not miss**
· Lumbar spine stress fracture · IV disc disease · Paraspinal myofascial tightness · Facet joint pathology · SIJ pathology	· IV disc prolapse · Spondylolisthesis · Joint hypermobility syndrome · Hip pathology · Seronegative spinal disease	· Malignancy · Spinal TB · Osteoporotic wedge fracture
IV, intervertebral; SIJ, sacroiliac joint; TB, tuberculosis.		

b. MRI is first-line imaging modality – early stress reactions appear as bone marrow oedema which appears as high intensity on T2WI. The presence of a complete fracture is difficult to establish on routine MRI sequences. More recent 3 Tesla (3T) MRI with thin-slice T1WI volumetric interpolated breath-hold examination (VIBE) sequence has also shown to have comparable accuracy to CT in the detection and characterisation of incomplete pars stress fractures

c. CT is useful to determine incomplete fractures, overall bony anatomy and assist in surgical planning

Classification: Hollenberg classification which is based on MRI features (1)

- Grade 0: Normal
- Grade I: Stress reaction indicated by marrow-oedema
- Grade II: Incomplete; thinning, fragmentation or irregularity of the pars visible on T1WI or T2WI
- Grade III: Acute complete stress fracture with marrow oedema; unilateral or bilateral
- Grade IV: Chronic defects indicated by a complete fracture but lack of marrow-oedema

Management: Average rehabilitation duration is 9 months. A simplified overview for rehabilitation of a pars interarticularis stress fracture in a fast bowler is shown in Figure 6.1.

1. Acute phase
   a. Education including explanation of plan for, and duration of, rehabilitation
   b. Relative reduction of load including avoidance of hyperextension or impact for at least 4 weeks
   c. Replace calcium and vitamin D if insufficient
   d. Analgesia
   e. Maintenance of cardiovascular (CV) fitness
   f. Strengthening exercises focussing on lumbopelvic control, e.g. squatting, lunging, bridges
   g. Continue to attend training if in an elite setting
   h. Advice on hamstring flexibility
   i. School bag advice – use a rucksack, avoid extremely heavy bags or bags over one shoulder
2. Subacute phase (when no rest pain and able to perform unloaded strengthening)
   a. Continue mobility and flexibility exercises
   b. CV fitness can include low impact activities, then jogging, and then progress to plyometrics
   c. Protected reloading including loaded strength exercises, e.g. dumbbell squats
   d. Sport-specific drills
3. Return to play (RTP) phase (when completion of strengthening programme without pain)
   a. Some clinicians like to see bony healing evident on repeat MRI
   b. Technique analysis and modification
   c. Gradual reintroduction to exacerbating activities, e.g. bowling or back hypertextension
   d. Return to training for minimum 1 week prior to RTP
   e. Elite: Daily clinical review and meeting with the multidisciplinary team (MDT)

If a chronic defect is present, the patient may benefit from a radiologically guided local anaesthetic (LA) injection.

ΔΔ: Facet joint pathology, spondylolisthesis, spondyloarthropathy (SpA)

SPONDYLOLISTHESIS

In the context of sporting injuries, and particularly in adolescents, spondylolisthesis is regarded as a continuum of disease secondary to a fracture of the pars interarticularis secondary to repetitive hyperextension. In adults an isthmic spondylolysis is common.

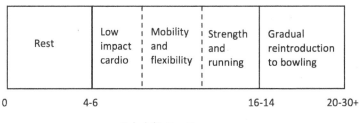

Rest	Low impact cardio	Mobility and flexibility	Strength and running	Gradual reintroduction to bowling

0   4-6   16-14   20-30+

Rehabilitation time
(weeks)

Figure 6.1 Overview of a simplified schema for rehabilitation of a pars interarticularis stress fracture in a fast bowler with approximate rehabilitation time in weeks.

Meyerding classification (2):

Grade I	<25%
Grade II	25–50%
Grade III	50–75%
Grade IV	>75%

Clinical features:

- Axial back pain especially on hyperextension
- Leg pain especially if L5 radiculopathy present

Investigations:

- X-ray: AP, lateral and oblique lumbar spine view to assess the degree of slip
- MRI to evaluate for foraminal stenosis

Management:

- Dependent on grade

- Conservative management as per spondylolysis if <50%
- Surgical referral if >50%, progressive slip or refractory pain to conservative management

LUMBAR DISC HERNIATION

Disc herniation is the displacement of intevertebral disc material beyond the normal confines of the disc and can be divided into protrusions or extrusions (Figure 6.2a). Lumbar disc herniation can cause a radicular pattern of lower back pain and leg pain, with 95% occurring between L4 and S1.

Disc herniation can be posterolateral (also known as paracentral; most common) or foraminal (Figure 6.2b).

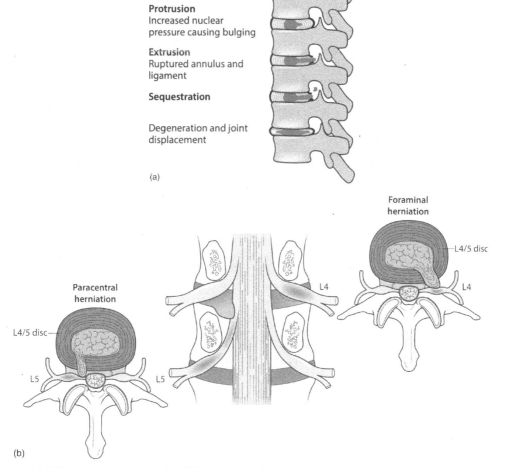

Figure 6.2 (a) Figure demonstrating the different types of disc herniation pathologies. (Reproduced with kind permission from *Apley & Solomon's System of Orthopaedics and Trauma*, 10th edition, CRC Press, 2018.) (b) Coronal and axial diagrams of paracentral and foraminal lumbar disc herniation.

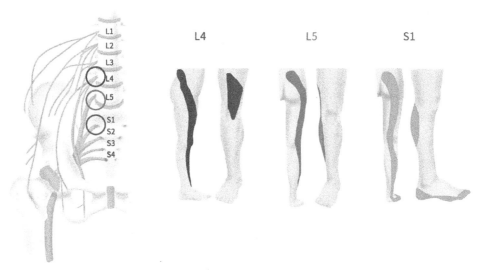

Figure 6.3 Pattern of lumbar radicular pain according to the level of the lesion.

- Posterolateral – affects the descending nerve root, e.g. L4/5 disc affects the L5 nerve root
- Foraminal – affects the exiting nerve root, e.g. L4/5 disc affects the L4 nerve root

Clinical features:

- Lower back pain
- Radicular pain, tingling and/or numbness in the distribution of the nerve root affected (Figure 6.3)
- May be accompanying motor weakness in corresponding myotomal distribution (Table 6.3)
- Cauda equina syndrome (see below)

Examination: see Table 6.3.

Investigations:

- MRI spine – sagittal T1WI images can provide the most diagnostic information. Once an abnormality has been detected, correlate these with the T2WI. Describe the appearance and the location of the abnormally displaced nucleus pulposus (3) (see Chapter 18).

Appearance:

- Protrusion: Focal herniation of disc material beyond the margins of the adjacent vertebral body, over <90° of circumference, with a base that is wider than dome
- Extrusion: Focal herniation of disc nuclear material through an annular defect, remaining in continuity with the disc, with a base narrower than the dome of the extrusion
- Sequestration: distal migration of extruded disc material away from the disc, with no direct continuation with the adjacent disc

Location (axial plane) and disc level (sagittal plane) should be described:

- Paracentral
- Subarticular
- Foraminal
- Extraforaminal
- Anterior

Management: the vast majority improve without surgical intervention:

- Analgesia – NSAIDs, e.g. naproxen

Table 6.3 Examination findings of lumbar radiculopathy according to the level of the lesion

	L3	L4	L5	S1
Sensory	Medial thigh	Medial foot	Between 1st and 2nd toe	Lateral foot
Motor	Hip flexion	Knee extension/ankle dorsiflexion	Ankle dorsiflexion/hallux dorsiflexion	Plantarflexion
Reflexes	–	Knee jerk	–	Ankle jerk
Other			SLR+ Slump+	SLR+ Slump+
SLR, straight leg raise				

- Relative rest and activity modification
- Strengthening programme
- If refractory, consider selective nerve root block or epidural or surgical referral for consideration of discectomy

Admit or refer urgently to orthopaedics or neurosurgeons if there is progressive, persistent, or severe neurological deficit.

ΔΔ: Hamstring muscle tear (e.g. L5), spinal stenosis, spondylolisthesis, infection, e.g. discitis, osteomyelitis, epidural abscess or malignancy, e.g. primary tumour or metastatic disease

CAUDA EQUINA SYNDROME

Cauda equina syndrome occurs secondary to compression of the nerve roots that originate from the conus medullaris at the base of the spinal cord.

Causes:

- Disc herniation (L4-L5 most common)
- Spinal stenosis
- Malignancy
- Trauma, e.g. lumbar burst fracture
- Epidural abscess
- Spinal epidural haematoma
- Spondylolisthesis

Clinical features and red flag symptoms:

- Bilateral sciatica
- Severe or progressive bilateral neurological deficit of the legs, such as major motor weakness with knee extension, ankle eversion or foot dorsiflexion
- Difficulty initiating micturition or impaired sensation of urinary flow, if untreated it may lead to urinary retention with overflow urinary incontinence
- Loss of sensation of rectal fullness, if untreated this may lead to fecal incontinence
- Perianal, perineal or genital sensory loss (saddle anaesthesia or paraesthesia)
- Reduced anal tone

In practice, anyone presenting with acute back pain and/or leg pain, with a suggestion of a disturbance of their bladder or bowel function and/or saddle sensory disturbance, should be suspected of having a cauda equina syndrome (4).

Examination: Full lower limb neurological and vascular examination should be performed

- Lower extremity weakness and sensory disturbance
- Reduced sensation to pinprick in perianal region (S2-4), perineum and posterior thigh
- Digital rectal exam: decreased rectal tone and diminished anal wink test

Investigations: Arrange urgent spinal MRI

- There should be a low threshold for investigation with an emergency scan
- Any reason for delay or decision not to perform should be clearly documented
- Ask patient to be nil by mouth until scan
- If confirmed, then immediate referral to spinal surgeons
- Bladder scan can be used to assess post-void residual volumes
- Blood workup if other aetiologies are expected, e.g. malignancy or abscess: FBC, U&E, CRP

Management is dependent on the underlying aetiology – urgent surgical decompression is normally undertaken. All patients should be safety-netted if presenting with back pain but not otherwise meeting criteria for an urgent scan.

LUMBAR SPINAL STENOSIS

This is a degenerative condition of the lumbar spine causing narrowing of the spinal canal secondary to either bony structures (e.g. facet or posterior vertebral body osteophytes or spondylolisthesis) or soft tissue structures (e.g. herniated disc, hypertrophy of ligamentum flavum). It is common in older males.

Clinical features:

- Lower back pain or leg pain
- Neurogenic claudication – pain worse with extension and relieved with flexion, e.g. will complain of pain walking downhill but relieved walking uphill. It is important to distinguish from vascular claudication which is relieved on stopping activity
- +/– weakness

Examination:

- May be normal
- Pain on back extension
- Reduced lumbar ROM especially in extension
- Perform full neurological examination – may be normal

Investigations:

- X-ray
  - AP and lateral views may show osteophytes or disc space narrowing
  - Flexion/extension views
- MRI can show canal stenosis and facet and ligament hypertrophy

Management:

- Conservative management includes analgesia, physiotherapy and corticosteroid injections

- Surgical options such as decompression are considered in those with symptoms refractory to conservative management

REFERENCES

1. Hollenberg GM, Beattie PF, Meyers SP, Weinberg EP, Adams MJ. Stress reactions of the lumbar pars interarticularis: The development of a new MRI classification system. *Spine (Phila Pa 1976)*. 2002;27(2):181–6.

2. Meyerding H. Spondyloptosis. *Surg Gynaecol Obstet*. 1932;54:371–7.

3. Fardon DF, Williams AL, Dohring EJ, Murtagh FR, Gabriel Rothman SL, Sze GK. Lumbar disc nomenclature: Version 2.0: Recommendations of the combined task forces of the North American Spine Society, the American Society of Spine Radiology and the American Society of Neuroradiology. *Spine J*. 2014;14:2525–45.

4. Surgeons TSoBN, Surgeons BAoS. *Standards of Care for Suspected and Confirmed Compressive Cauda Equina Syndrome*, 2018.

HIP

The key differential diagnoses of the hip are summarised in Table 7.1.

FEMOROACETABULAR IMPINGEMENT (FAI)

FAI is a clinical syndrome characterised by painful, limited hip motion secondary to underlying morphological variants of the femoral head/neck region and/or acetabulum. These morphological variants are Cam, pincer and mixed (Table 7.2 and Figure 7.1).

Clinical features:

- Groin and/or hip pain
- Limited hip range of movement (ROM)
- Mechanical symptoms if labral involvement

Examination:

- Restricted hip ROM, particularly internal rotation (IR) with the hip flexed
- FADIR +

Investigations:

- X-ray: Anterior posterior (AP) and true lateral (15° IR) views, Dunn view (patient supine with hip flexed to 90° and abducted 20° with a neutral pelvis)
  - Calculate alpha angle on lateral X-ray for Cam deformity by measuring the angle between the orientation of the femoral neck and the margin of the femoral head
- Magnetic resonance imaging (MRI) +/− arthrography to assess labrum

Management:

- Conservative: Activity modification, movement retraining, analgesia

- Surgical referral if persistent and debilitating symptoms or mechanical symptoms. Options include arthroscopic labral repair, osteochondroplasty or open periacetabular osteotomy

FEMORAL NECK STRESS FRACTURE

"A 35-year-old amateur female runner presents with anterior thigh pain after recently taking up road running. She is currently training for her first half marathon which she is running for charity and she works as a teacher. She has a BMI of 19 and is vegan."

Explore potential causes in history and examination including:

a. Training load
b. Nutritional and menstrual history
c. Biomechanical abnormalities

Clinical features:

- Dull, poorly localised ache in anterior thigh, which can radiate to the groin or knee
- Commonly seen in distance runners

Examination:

- Pain on palpation anterior hip or greater trochanter
- Hop test +
- Assess leg length and alignment
- Fulcrum test +

Investigations:

- Blood tests: Full blood count (FBC), urea and electrolytes (U&E), liver function tests (LFTs), bone profile, vitamin D, thyroid function tests (TFTs) and consider phosphate (PO_4^{2-}),

DOI: 10.1201/9781003163701-9

Table 7.1 Differential diagnosis of hip pathology according to location

Anterior	Lateral	Posterior
FAI or labral pathology	Gluteus medius pathology	Posterior labral tear
Stress fracture NOF	Trochanteric bursa	Referred from lumbar spine or pelvis
Traction apophysitis (ASIS/AIIS)	Stress fracture NOF	Proximal hamstring
Avascular necrosis		Sciatic nerve entrapment
Slipped upper femoral epiphysis		
Transient osteoporosis		

ASIS, anterior superior iliac spine; AIIS, anterior inferior iliac spine; FAI, femoroacetabular impingement; NOF, neck of femur.

Table 7.2 Morphological and radiological features associated with Cam and pincer lesions in FAI

Cam	Pincer
• Reduced head to neck ratio • Reduced femoral offset • Associated with previous SUFE or Legg-Calve-Perthes (Perthes) disease • X-ray: Pistol grip deformity, alpha angle > 50°, head-neck offset ratio on lateral X-ray < 0.17	• Acetabular rim overhang • Associated with acetabular protrusion, acetabular retroversion and coxa profundal • X-ray: Crossover sign (acetabular retroversion)

SUFE, superior upper femoral epiphysis.

parathyroid hormone (PTH), ferritin and iron studies, anti-TTG for coeliac screen and sex hormones
- Imaging:
  - X-ray if >6 weeks
  - MRI will show bone marrow oedema on T2WI
  - Dual-energy X-ray absorptiometry (DEXA) scan if features of relative energy deficiency in sport (RED-S)

Management: Should include addressing risk factors and also depends on whether the stress fracture is superior (tensile) or inferior (compression-sided; Figure 7.2)

Management for inferior (compression-sided) femoral neck stress fractures

1. Offload with activity modification and relative rest +/− crutch if pain on weight bearing (WB)
2. Analgesia (not non-steroidal anti-inflammatories [NSAIDs] as can impair bony healing)
3. Address underlying cause:
   a. Education regarding training load progression, e.g. increase by <10% per week
   b. Biomechanical correction – encourage forefoot strike if distance runner and increase cadence
   c. Nutritional analysis with dietician if necessary

HEALTHY HIP JOINT

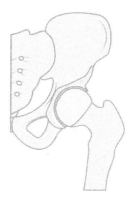

MIXED FEMOROACETABULAR IMPINGEMENT (FAI)

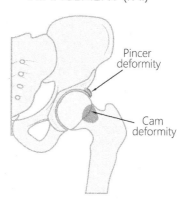

Pincer deformity

Cam deformity

Figure 7.1 Illustration of a Cam pincer and mixed morphology in FAI.

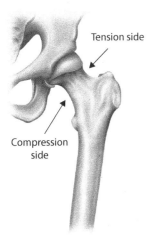

Figure 7.2 Femoral neck stress fractures. Tension (*superior*) side and compression (*inferior*) side.

4. Optimise lifestyle measures, e.g. stop smoking, dietary advice if under-fuelling and consider vitamin D supplementation (supplement if deficient <30 nmol/L or insufficient 30–50 nmol/L with 4000 IU daily)
5. Maintain ROM and cardiovascular (CV) fitness – swim, cycle, upper body strength and trunk stability
6. Graded rehabilitation programme
   a. Muscle strengthening – pelvis and lower limbs
   b. Return to running when single leg press 1.5× body weight
7. Return to play (RTP) governed by clinical assessment of pain, strength and ROM
8. Address psychological aspects and involve multidisciplinary team (MDT) if in an elite setting including coach, dietician and psychologist

Management for superior (tension-sided) femoral stress fractures

1. Offload and surgical referral given high risk of non-union

LATERAL HIP PAIN

Common differentials which overlap include:

- Gluteal tendinopathy
- Proximal iliotibial band (ITB) syndrome
- Greater trochanteric pain syndrome (GTPS)

Gluteal tendinopathy / GTPS

Gluteal tendinopathy is thought to be secondary to compression of gluteus medius +/– minimus tendon or bursae between greater trochanter and the ITB.

Clinical features:

- Aching around the greater trochanter which can radiate down the ITB or into the groin or buttock
- Pain when running on camber, running uphill or during single leg weight bearing
- Pain when lying on the affected side

Examination:

- Tenderness over gluteus medius insertion at the lateral aspect of the greater trochanter
- Pain and/or weakness on resisted hip abduction
- FABER+
- May be Trendelenberg +
- Usually normal hip ROM
- May be Ober's test +

Investigations:

- Normally a clinical diagnosis
- Ultrasound (US) or MRI can help to confirm – US may show thickening of tendon or hypoechoic changes +/– changes in the bursa. It is important to rule out a tear of the tendon which may limit potential adjunctive treatments you can offer.
- If diagnosis unclear whether coming from lateral hip or intra-articular, consider diagnostic steroid + local anaesthetic (LA) injection.

Management:

- Stop provoking activities, e.g. running on a camber or uphill, sitting with knees crossed or sleeping on the affected side
- Progressive loading programme:
  - Isometrics of hip abductors, e.g. push knee against wall when standing next to a wall
  - TheraBand™ hip abduction exercise
  - Isotonic movements, e.g. sliders into abduction or bridges
  - Progress to more functional movements, e.g. double leg squat and straight line running
- Technique analysis:
  - Increase cadence and reduce stride length
  - Landing correction
- Consider extra-corporal shock wave therapy (ESWT) if refractory and no evidence of a tear

BUTTOCK PAIN

PROXIMAL HAMSTRING ORIGIN TENDINOPATHY

This is common in sprinters and long-distance runners, secondary to overuse or an acute tear where the hamstring tendons originate from the ischial tuberosity. It commonly co-exists with ischiogluteal bursitis.

Examination:

- Pain on hamstring stretch
- Tenderness over the ischial tuberosity on direct palpation

Investigations:

- US or MRI. MRI may show increased tendon size, peritendinous T2WI signal and ischial tuberosity oedema

Management:

- Analgesia, advise against prolonged sitting
- Continue CV fitness, e.g. stationary cycling
- Staged progressive loading:
  - Isometric contractions, e.g. hamstring curl prone or supine bridge for 60 seconds, 3–5 reps, aiming for a visual analogue scale (VAS) ≤ 4/10
  - Isotonic exercises, e.g. bridging on a gym ball (double then progress to single leg), Romanian deadlifts and single leg squats
  - Progress to Nordic hamstring exercises
  - Running drills then progress to plyometric exercises, e.g. jumping, hopping, change of direction, sprinting
- Technique analysis, e.g. shorter stride

HAMSTRING MUSCLE INJURY

Injuries to the muscles of the hamstring commonly occur in biceps femoris. They can generally be divided into type 1 and type 2 injuries (Table 7.3).

Clinical features:

- Sudden onset pain or a 'pop' felt in the back of the leg and buttock
- Symptoms of mild injuries may only appear the following day

Examination:

- Antalgic gait
- Tender to palpation over the affected muscle
- Hamstring stretch +
- Bruising or swelling
- Assess for biomechanical risk factors during examination including pelvic anteversion (lordosis+) or tight quadriceps (modified Thomas' test; knee extension)

Table 7.3 Differences in types 1 and 2 hamstring muscle injuries

Type 1	Type 2
High-speed running	Stretch type injury
Long head of biceps femoris	Close to ischial tuberosity
Proximal muscle tendon junction	Proximal free tendon of semimembranosus

- Ensure lumbar spine examination is clear

Investigations:

- MRI is the gold standard investigation which may demonstrate hyperintensity of the injured area suggesting oedema. Most commonly this is in the musculotendinous junction (see Chapter 18). The optimal time to perform the scan has been reported as between 48 to 96 hours post-injury (1).
- US can also be used
  Determine the size of the injury and the location, e.g. origin, proximal free tendon, myotendinous junction (biceps femoris common), myofascial, intramuscular, distal free tendon (semitendinosus most common). Note: Bleeding around the sciatic nerve can cause prolonged symptoms.
- If an avulsion is suspected, then X-rays may be useful

British Athletics Injury classification (2):

- Myofascial
- Musculotendinous junction (MTJ)
- Intratendinous

Grade according to the extent of oedema or architectural disruption:

- Small tear
- Moderate tear
- Extensive tear
- Complete tear

Management: Criteria-dependent progression

As a general rule of thumb return to play times are as follows:

Muscle	3 weeks
MTJ	6 weeks
Intratendinous	9+ weeks – delay eccentric training by 3 weeks

Note: Injury to the intramuscular conjoint tendon of the long head of biceps femoris, proximal MTJ of biceps tendon and the distal tendon junction of biceps femoris are associated with a prolonged recovery.

Acute phase

- Protect, ice, optimal loading, compression, elevation (POLICE), analgesia
- Muscle activation 3–4×/day, low grade pain-free, e.g. prone knee bends
- Aim for pain-free walking and restore ROM
- Maintain CV fitness throughout, e.g. rowing, stationary cycle, stepper

Can progress to the next stage when walking pain-free and isometrics can be performed pain-free

Subacute phase

- Muscle strengthening
  - Muscle strengthening of hamstrings, 3 sets of 12 repetitions:
    - e.g. extender, diver, glider, TheraBand™ exercises
    - Bridges
    - Single leg roll out on a Swiss ball
    - Nordic hamstring exercises (high eccentric element so only do this late in rehabilitation)
    - Deadlifts
    - Delay eccentric exercises until later in rehabilitation, especially if tendon involvement
  - Muscle strengthening of synergists, i.e. gluteus maximus, adductor magnus
    - Squats, deep lunge
  - Neuromuscular (NM) control – proprioceptive exercises on BOSU

Progress when can perform the above pain free, with good form and no guarding

2. Functional exercises
   - Return to running programme
   - Sport-specific drills, e.g. fast feet
3. Maintain CV fitness throughout
4. Attend training and address risk factors, e.g. muscle weakness or imbalances

Progress to training when minimal symptoms and a return to running programme has been completed, there is full and pain free ROM and athlete is able to perform the Askling H test.

Return to play phase: *Return to play once completed one week of full training*

GROIN PAIN

"A 25-year-old elite footballer is struggling with a 5-month history of groin pain, worse when kicking. There is no history of a traumatic or inciting event. Please assess."

Longstanding groin pain should be defined using the *Doha* agreement (3) (Table 7.4). Pain can either be an acute strain or an overuse injury.

Investigations:

- X-ray: Degenerative changes of the symphyseal joint
- Ultrasound: Adductor muscle insertion pathology
- +/− MRI: Pubic-related pain to look for bone marrow oedema and secondary cleft signs

ADDUCTOR-RELATED GROIN PAIN

Clinical features:

- Medial groin pain where adductor longus attaches onto the pubic bone, which can also radiate down the inner thigh
- Pain during sprinting and kicking are also common complaints

Examination:

- Tender to palpation where adductor longus attaches to the pubic bone
- Adductor squeeze test +

Management:

Acute phase
- Relative offloading by stopping aggravating activity, e.g. kicking
- POLICE if acute strain
- Isometric exercise, e.g. adduction with ball between knees supine for 30 seconds (10 sets with 30 seconds recovery)
- Adduct until the point of pain aiming for pain <3/10

Progress when isometrics does not cause pain and ROM >50% compared with uninjured side

Conditioning phase
- Introduce dynamic adduction exercise with low load and high reps, e.g. TheraBand™ adduction, side lying with adduction
- Also condition hip flexors and abdominals
  - Gradually increase load and reduce repetitions
  - Increase complexity and proprioception, e.g. exercises on Swiss ball

Table 7.4 Clinical features and return to play time according to groin injury region as per the Doha agreement

Region	Diagnostic clinical features	RTP time
Adductor	Adductor tenderness AND pain on resisted adductor testing	6–12/52
Iliopsoas	Pain on resisted hip flexion AND/OR pain on stretching the hip flexors	4–6
Inguinal	Pain in inguinal canal and tenderness of the inguinal canal; no palpable inguinal hernia. More likely if aggravated by abdominal resistance or Valsalva/cough/sneeze	8–12
Pubic	Local tenderness of pubic symphysis and immediately adjacent bone	12
RTP, return to play		

Progress when minimal adductor guarding, minimal pain on resisted exercises, ROM 80%

Sport-specific phase
- Progressive return to running and kicking programme
  - Starting with straight line running, then lateral running, backwards running
  - Gradually increase duration and then intensity
- High-level Copenhagen hip adductor exercises
- Introduce kicking and ball or passing skills

Progress when no guarding, minimal pain on exercises, ROM 100%, strength > 80%

Return to play
- Non-contact training, then progress to contact training
- At least one week of full contact training prior to return to match play

ILIOPSOAS-RELATED GROIN PAIN

Clinical features: Pain tends to be located in the proximal thigh anteriorly and sometimes can be in the lower abdomen.

Examination:

- Pain on resisted hip flexion or on passive stretch
- Pain on palpation
- Hip flexion when performing modified Thomas' test

Management:

Acute phase
- Relative offloading by stopping aggravating activity, e.g. running
- Isometric exercises, e.g. hold hip in flexion by sitting on a chair and pushing hand against knee
- 30 second holds (10 reps with 30 seconds recovery)
- Pelvic stabilisation, e.g. two leg bridges

Progress when isometrics does not cause pain and ROM >50% compared with uninjured side

Conditioning phase
- Introduce isotonic exercise with low load and high reps, e.g. TheraBand™ hip flexion, two leg hip thrusters, abdominal exercises
- Gradually increase load and reduce repetitions, e.g. aim for three sets of eight repetitions with fatigue in the final repetition
- Increase complexity and proprioception, e.g. one leg hip thruster, forward lunges, squats on unstable surface, e.g. BOSU ball, one leg Romanian dead lift

Progress when minimal guarding, minimal pain on resisted exercises, ROM 80%

Sport-specific phase
- Progressive return to running and kicking programme
  - Starting with straight line running, then lateral running, backwards running
  - Gradually increase duration and then intensity
- High level eccentric hip flexion exercises
- Introduce kicking and ball or passing skills

Progress when no guarding, minimal pain on exercises, ROM 100%, strength > 80%

Return to play
- Non-contact training then progress to contact training
- At least one week of full contact training prior to return to match play

INGUINAL-RELATED GROIN PAIN

Inguinal-related groin pain can be attributed to a number of anatomical structures, including the rectus abdominus, internal oblique, transversalis muscles or conjoint tendon at the pubic tubercle.

Clinical features:

- Pain experienced deep in the groin, more proximal than adductor-related pain. Pain is diffuse with possible radiation along the inguinal ligament, perineum or rectus muscles
- Tenderness at the conjoint tendon
- Tenderness at the external ring of the inguinal canal
- Pain with increased abdominal pressure, e.g. coughing
- +/− dilatation of the external ring, but in the absence of a true hernia

Management: As per adductor- and iliopsoas-related pain, but rehabilitation may take longer.

PUBIC-RELATED GROIN PAIN

Clinical features:

- Central groin pain with localised tenderness at the pubic symphysis
- No specialised test can reliably differentiate from other diagnoses

Investigations:

- If longstanding, X-ray can demonstrate erosions of the pubic symphysis with sclerosis and osteophyte formation. MRI can demonstrate increased signal around the symphysis.

Management:

- As per adductor- and iliopsoas-related pain
- Poor evidence based on current best management

ΔΔ:

- Nerve entrapment including the ilioinguinal, genitofemoral or lateral femoral cutaneous nerves
- Stress fracture of NOF or inferior pubic ramus
- Avulsion fractures in adolescents
- Inguinal hernia
- Scrotal abnormalities, e.g. epididymitis, torsion, varicocele, hydrocele
- Referred pain from abdominal viscera, e.g. appendicitis, ectopic pregnancy, ovarian cyst, urinary tract infection (UTI) or lithiasis

ANTERIOR THIGH PAIN

Differential diagnoses of anterior thigh pain include:

- Quadriceps muscle injury
- Stress fracture of the femur
- Femoral nerve injury
- Nerve entrapment, e.g. lateral femoral cutaneous nerve
- Slipped upper femoral epiphysis (SUFE)
- Perthes' disease
- Avulsion of the anterior inferior iliac spine (AIIS; rectus femoris direct head)
- Myositis ossificans
- Malignancy, e.g. osteosarcoma

QUADRICEPS MUSCLE INJURY

Common sites are the distal portion of the MTJ of rectus femoris or the proximal rectus femoris (longer to heal).

Clinical features:

- Pain with muscle stretch
- Tender to palpation, usually laterally or distally
- Depending on grade, loss of strength

Investigations:

- X-ray: Useful to rule out other pathology, e.g. avulsion
- US: May show defect in the muscle or MTJ +/− haematoma
- MRI: This is the most sensitive modality which will show increased signal on T2WI within the muscle, MTJ or tendon

Management:

Acute phase
- Relative rest
- POLICE

- Analgesia (avoiding NSAIDs in first 72 hours)
- ROM exercises and gait exercises
- Quadriceps setting exercises, e.g. push knee into bed whilst supine

Progress when gait normal, isometric contraction pain-free and ROM >50% compared with unaffected side

Conditioning phase
- Introduce isotonic exercise with low load and high reps, e.g. TheraBand™ knee extension, squats against wall
- Gradually increase load and reduce repetitions, e.g. double leg squat, lunges, hip hikes
- Increase complexity and proprioception, e.g. single leg squat, weighted lunges

Progress when minimal guarding, minimal pain on resisted exercises, ROM 80%

Sport-specific phase
- Progressive return to running programme
- Starting with straight line running, then lateral running, backwards running, hops, change of direction
- Gradually increase duration and then intensity
- Sport specific drills, e.g. passing, dribbling

Progress when no guarding, minimal pain on exercises, ROM 100%, strength >80%

Return to Play
- Non-contact training then progress to contact training
- At least one week of full contact training prior to return to match play

MYOSITIS OSSIFICANS CIRCUMSCRIPTA

This condition is characterised by non-neoplastic heterotopic bone formation following a traumatic injury, commonly a blunt injury in large muscles of the extremities.

Clinical features:

- Tender swelling presenting following traumatic injury
- +/− restricted ROM, commonly over the diaphysis of long bones

Investigations:

- X-rays demonstrate opacification with periosteal calcification (see Chapter 18).
- CT or MRI can provide further bony and soft tissue differentiation. The main differential is malignancy, so this should be ruled out.

Management: The majority of cases resolve spontaneously but may require active monitoring until cessation

REFERENCES

1. Slavotinek JP, Verrall GM, Fon GT. Hamstring injury in athletes: Using MR imaging measurements to compare extent of muscle injury with amount of time lost from competition. *AJR Am J Roentgenol*. 2002;179(6):1621–8.

2. Pollock N, James SL, Lee JC, Chakraverty R. British athletics muscle injury classification: A new grading system. *Br J Sports Med*. 2014;48:1347–51. England: Published by the BMJ Publishing Group Limited.

3. Weir A, Brukner P, Delahunt E, Ekstrand J, Griffin D, Khan KM, et al. Doha Agreement meeting on terminology and definitions in groin pain in athletes. *Br J Sports Med*. 2015;49(12):768–74.

8 Knee and leg

KNEE

ACUTE INJURIES

"An 18-year-old national female footballer has attended your clinic 7 days after sustaining an acute injury to their left knee, after which they were unable to weight bear. Please take a history and examine this patient."

ANTERIOR CRUCIATE LIGAMENT (ACL) TEAR

Mechanism of injury: non-contact valgus force with torsion or hyperextension common during cutting or pivoting

Clinical features:

- Immediately painful
- May have heard a 'pop' when it occurred
- Unable to continue activity
- +/− haemarthrosis

Examination:

- Acutely can be very swollen so often difficult to examine
- Reduced range of movement (ROM)
- Effusion
- Lateral joint tenderness,
- Special tests: Lachman test+, anterior drawer+
- If associated meniscal injury, then McMurray's +

Investigations:

- X-ray: Rule out Segond fracture or tibial plateau fracture. You may see deepening of the lateral sulcus terminalis.

- Magnetic Resonance Imaging (MRI):
  - Sagittal view: Discontinuity of tendon fibres on T2WI, tendon that does not align with Blumensaat's line, associated bone oedema (typical pattern from pivot shift type injury is contracoup bone marrow oedema on lateral femoral condyle and posterolateral tibia)
  - Coronal: 'Empty notch' sign on T1WI (see 'chapter 18)
  - Can also detect associated injuries (meniscal, medial collateral ligament [MCL], posterolateral corner [PLC] injury) which will guide management

Management: Operative versus non-operative/conservative (see 'Clinical Management Stations' chapter 12 for discussion)

Conservative management:
- Rehabilitation is milestone driven but on average return to play (RTP) is approximately 6–9 months

  Acute phase:
  - Activity modification and analgesia
  - ROM exercises – heel slides, sitting passive leg extension and flexion (use other leg)
  - Quadriceps isometric exercises (plus hamstring and calf isometric exercises)
  - Body weight exercises supine – gentle straight leg raise (SLR), hip abduction
  - Gait exercises
  - May require brace plus crutches during this period

Progress when full active extension and 120° active flexion, little effusion and can hold terminal extension in single leg standing, pain-free walking

DOI: 10.1201/9781003163701-10

Reconditioning phase:

- Muscle strengthening – leg press 0–30°, mini squats, calf raise, hamstring curls
  - Progress to lunges, step ups and bridges and from two to one leg, lateral movement
- Maintain cardiovascular (CV) fitness – stationary bicycle, elliptical trainer
- Proprioception exercises – single leg stance, tandem walking, progress difficulty with wobble board
- Introduce movement, e.g. forward lunge walk, lateral stepping

Progress when full ROM, able to perform exercises with no pain

Sport-specific/functional phase:

- Return to running programme – when can perform single less press 1.5× body weight (BW)
  - Progress to arabesque, jumping, hopping and changing direction with jumping and landing drills
- Re-educate landing mechanics and instigate prevention programme including strength and conditioning (S&C) programme

RTP when single leg hop >90% contralateral

ΔΔ: Patellar dislocation

POSTERIOR CRUCIATE LIGAMENT (PCL) TEAR

Mechanism of injury: Falling on bent knee, hyperextension of bent knee, dashboard injury. Posterior cruciate ligament injuries are rarely isolated, and they commonly involve posterolateral corner (PLC) injuries (see Table 8.1 for contents of PLC).

Table 8.1 Major static and dynamic stabilisers of posterolateral corner

Contents of the posterolateral corner	
Major static stabilisers	**Dynamic stabilisers**
Popliteus tendon	Biceps femoris
LCL	Popliteus muscle
Popliteofibular	ITB
ligament	Lateral head of
	gastrocnemius

ITB, iliotibial band; LCL, lateral collateral ligament.

Clinical features:

- Poorly defined pain
- Swelling
- Feeling of instability

Examination:

- Associated with less swelling than ACL
- Posterior sag +
- Posterior drawer test +
- +/− positive dial test if associated PLC injury

Investigations:

- X-ray: Anteroposterior (AP) and lateral views
- Stress radiograph: Assess for posterior translation of tibia
- MRI: High signal within ligament, disrupted ligament, enlarged and swollen PCL >7 mm AP diameter of vertical tendon. Also assess for bone contusion of the posterior margin of the femoral condyle or the posterior tibial condyle (see Chapter 18)

Classification is based on the position of the medial tibial plateau in relation to medial femoral condyle at 90° flexion

- Grade 1 <0.5 cm
- Grade 2 0.5–1 cm
- Grade 3 >1 cm

Management:

- If the injury is isolated, then management can be conservative with an extension brace for 2 weeks (RTP approximately 6–10 weeks)
- Surgical referral if instability and/or PLC injury

PATELLAR DISLOCATION

Mechanism of injury: Mechanism can be traumatic (commonly quadriceps contraction with sudden flexion and external rotation of the tibia) or as part of a clinical picture associated with hypermobility. Normally there is disruption to medial patellofemoral ligament (MPFL).

Risk factors for patellar dislocation are summarised in Table 8.2.

Clinical features:

- Immediate swelling and pain
- 'Pop' sensation
- Difficulty weight bearing
- Some may report seeing the patella move out of place

Table 8.2 Risk factors for patellar dislocation

| General | Anatomical | |
	Bony	Muscle
• Hypermobility • Previous dislocation • Increased Q angle – associated with genu valgum, pronated feet	• Patellar alta • Trochlear dysplasia • Increased TT-TG distance	• Weak medial musculature • Overpull of lateral structures including VL or ITB

ITB, iliotibial band; TT-TG, tibial tubercle to trochlear groove; VL, vastus lateralis.

Examination:

- Effusion
- Lateral apprehension test +
- Pain on quadriceps contraction
- Tender over medial patellar border (MPFL)

Investigations:

- X-ray: AP, lateral, sunrise views to assess bony anatomy for risk factors or osteochondral fragment
  - Lateral: Trochlear dysplasia (crossing sign or double contour sign) and patellar height (Insall-Salvati 0.8–1.2)
  - Sunrise view: Lateral patellar tilt (lateral patellofemoral [PF] angle normally >11°)
- Computed tomography (CT): Calculate tibial tubercle-trochlear groove (TT-TG) distance (>20 mm normal)
- MRI: Bone oedema on inferomedial patella and lateral femoral condyle (see Chapter 18)

Management:

- Conservative: Address risk factors, rehabilitation should focus on strengthening medial structures. May need extension splint (RTP 8–12 weeks)
- Surgical referral if an osteochondral lesion, substantial disruption of medial patellar stabilisers, recurrent dislocations or if symptoms are refractory to rehabilitation

MEDIAL AND LATERAL COLLATERAL LIGAMENT INJURY

Medial collateral ligament injury

Mechanism of injury: Direct blow to the outside of the knee, or outward twisting of knee with the foot planted. It can be injured in association with an ACL injury and medial meniscus tear.

Clinical features:

- Medial sided knee pain, medial sided swelling, mild effusion

Examination:

- Effusion
- Tender over MCL
- Pain or laxity on valgus stress at 30° flexion
- Assess for saphenous nerve injury:
  - Paraesthesia in the infrapatellar region

Investigations:

- X-ray: To exclude a fracture
- MRI: Discontinuity or wavy ligament and high signal intensity on T2WI. Most injuries of the MCL are at the femoral attachment.

Management: The majority of isolated low-grade injuries can be treated conservatively with a progressive rehabilitation programme and some may require a brace initially. The average RTP is 8 weeks for an isolated injury.

Lateral collateral ligament injury

Mechanism of injury: Direct blow to the medial side of the knee, hyperextension stress, any varus loading of knee. Can be associated with cruciate ligament injuries or injuries to the posterolateral corner.

Clinical features:

- Lateral joint line pain
- Swelling
- Instability

Examination:

- Tender over insertion on the fibular head
- Pain or laxity on varus stress at 30° flexion
- Dial test for PLC
- Assess for peroneal nerve injury: Paraesthesia in the top of the foot or outer part of the lower leg

Investigations:

- X-ray: Rule out a fracture
- MRI: Discontinuity or high signal in tendon on T2WI and to assess for associated injuries

Management: Isolated low-grade injuries with no instability can be treated conservatively with a progressive rehabilitation programme

MENISCAL INJURIES

Mechanism of injury: Acute injuries tend to be secondary to a twisting injury, often injured alongside ACL. The medial meniscus is more commonly injured compared with the lateral meniscus due to its attachment to the medical joint capsule and MCL which makes it relatively less mobile. Chronic degenerative meniscus lesions may not have a preceding acute injury.

Clinical features:

- Pain in either medial or lateral joint line,
- Mechanical symptoms, e.g. locking, joint effusion.

Examination:

- Joint line tenderness
- Pain on 'duckwalking', i.e. hyperflexion of the knee joint
- Special tests: McMurray's +, Thessaly test +, Apley grind +

Investigations:

- X-ray: First line to look for other pathology, e.g. acute fracture
- MRI: May demonstrate high signal in the meniscus which extends to at least one articular surface, distortion of meniscal morphology, double PCL sign if bucket handle tear (see Chapter 18)

Types: Longitudinal, flap, radial, bucket handle, horizontal cleavage, degenerative

Management:

- Treatment depends on the location (vascularisation), position and pattern and age of patient
- First-line treatment is conservative management with education and rehabilitation
- Poor candidates for surgery include degenerative lesions, horizontal cleavage and complex tears. Partial meniscectomy has been shown to be no better than sham surgery for degenerative tears (1)
- Good candidates for meniscal repair include bucket handle tears, tears in the outer (red-red) zone (good vascularisation), <4 cm length, vertical or longitudinal tear. Partial meniscectomy considered for complex or radial patterns.

ΔΔ: Articular cartilage lesions – these generally have a more insidious onset and may have intermittent pain and swelling.

CHRONIC KNEE PAIN

Location of knee pain is important in determining differentials of chronic knee pain (Figure 8.1 and Table 8.3).

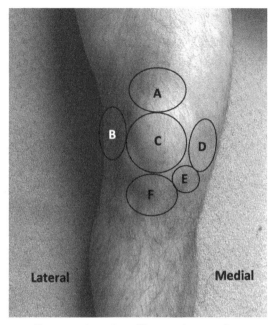

Figure 8.1 Location of knee pain according to different 'zones' can help narrow down the differential diagnosis.

Table 8.3 Differential diagnosis of chronic knee pain according to location of pain

Zone	Differentials
A	• Quadriceps tendinopathy
B	• Iliotibial band syndrome • Lateral meniscus tear • LCL injury
C	• Patellofemoral pain syndrome • Chrondromalacia patellae • Osteoarthritis • Prepatellar bursitis
D	• Medial meniscus tear • MCL injury • Osteoarthritis
E	• Pes anserine bursitis • Medial plica syndrome
F	• Patellar tendinopathy • Osgood-Schlatter disease • Sinding-Larsen-Johansson • Osteochondritis dissecans

LCL, lateral collateral ligament; MCL, medial collateral ligament.

Anterior knee pain

"This 40-year-old woman has been referred by her General Practitioner (GP) with pain in the front of her patellae bilaterally, aggravated by going up and down stairs. Please take a history and examination and explain any investigations and management you would recommend."

Key points in the history, in particular to differentiate patellofemoral pain (PFP) and patellar tendinopathy (PT):

- Initial onset of pain
- Specific location of pain
- Precise aggravating activities
- Change in load
- Any associated clicking or swelling

PATELLOFEMORAL PAIN SYNDROME

Clinical features:

- Vague ache anterior knee
- Symptoms aggravated by downhill running, stairs, squatting or prolonged sitting
- Clicking or 'grating' behind patella

Examination:

- Tenderness behind patella or infrapatellar
- +/− crepitus and effusion
- Squinting patellae, pronated feet, tibial torsion
- Pelvic drop in single leg squat

Investigations: Clinical diagnosis, US can help differentiate between patellar tendinopathy. You can assess bony anatomy for predisposing factors such as trochlear dysplasia or TT-TG distance.

Management:

1. Reduce pain – avoid aggravating activities (e.g. lunges or deep squats), analgesia, ice
2. Address extrinsic risk factors, e.g. training load, shoes, surface, orthoses if required, tight muscles
3. Patellar mobilisation of soft tissues if tight lateral structures
4. Taping, e.g. medial glide
5. Rehabilitation
   a. Prone and standing quadriceps stretch
   b. Quadriceps strengthening – isometrics, SLR, double leg squat and step ups with technique pointers (knee over toes)
   c. Hip and external rotation (ER) strengthening – control of pelvis during dynamic movement
   d. Kinetic chain strengthening
   e. Progress to plyometrics – power jumps with landing technique pointers
   f. Technique adjustment

PATELLAR TENDINOPATHY

Clinical features:

- Pain inferior pole of patella,
- Commonly aggravated by jumping.
- Pain may 'warm up' during training session.
- Rarely crepitus or an effusion

Examination:

- May be thickened tendon
- Pain on palpation of the inferior pole patella

Investigations: Not always necessary

- US: Hypoechoic changes, thickened tendon, neovascularisation
- MRI: Increased signal in tendon at proximal end

Management:

- Activity modification to reduce load – reduce aggravating activities, e.g. jumping and landing or reduce overall weekly training hours
- Address biomechanical drivers, e.g. assess landing technique – forefoot landing preferred
- Rehabilitation focussed on progressive loading of the tendon – RTP 6+ months, aim for pain <4/10 during exercises and no significant flare the next day
  - Isometric contractions – 45 seconds ×5, e.g. on leg extension machine
  - Isotonic exercises – squat three sets of 15 reps with isometrics before, twice per day
  - Progress to heavier load (heavy slow resistance), e.g. single leg press, squat on decline board. Three sets of 15 repetitions, then progress load to six repetitions with 2 mins rest, 3×/week
  - Progress to energy storage when can single leg press 1.5× body weight, e.g. lunges
  - Progress to sport specific, e.g. jumping, change direction
- Evidence is mixed regarding injection therapies and extra-corporal shock wave therapy (ESWT)

Note: If in season, avoid heavy eccentric loading, e.g. decline board.

ΔΔ: Infrapatellar fat pad impingement, synovial plica

OSTEOCHONDRITIS DISSECANS

Separation of an osteochondral fragment with gradual fragmentation of the articular surface, resulting in an osteochondral defect. It can be associated with intra-articular loose bodies.

Classically described on the lateral aspect of the medical epicondyle (LAME).

Clinical features:

- Vague activity-related pain
- Effusion
- Mechanical symptoms

Examination: Joint line tenderness, effusion

> ### Clanton classification
>
> Type I   – Depressed osteochondral fracture
> Type II – Fragment attached by osseous bridge
> Type III – Detached but non-displaced fragment
> Type IV – Displaced fragment

Staging: Clanton classification (see the box titled 'Clanton classification')

Investigations:

- X-ray: (AP, lateral and notch view) may miss early changes. Assess for subtle flattening or indistinct radiolucency around the cortical surface or frank fragmentation
- MRI: High signal between fragment and adjacent bone on T2WI, cysts beneath lesion, a focal osteochondral defect indicates detachment of the fragment (see Chapter 18)

Management:

- Offloading with relative rest and rehabilitation
- Surgical referral if fragment displaced or unstable

EXERCISE-INDUCED LEG PAIN

"You have been referred an 18-year-old infantryman from your local defence rehabilitation centre. He has developed pain in his shins, right worse than left, during his recent basic training and the pain is worse when running and immediately after. Please assess."

COMMON DIFFERENTIAL DIAGNOSES

- Bone stress: Stress reaction/fracture or medial tibial stress syndrome (MTSS)
- Chronic exertional compartment syndrome (CECS)
- Popliteal artery entrapment syndrome (PAES)
- Peripheral nerve entrapment, e.g. common peroneal nerve, superficial peroneal nerve, saphenous nerve
- Lumbar radiculopathy
- Other: Deep vein thrombosis (DVT), tibialis anterior tendinopathy, muscle injury, referred pain from knee, spinal stenosis

Note: If athlete has recently returned from training camp or competition abroad and had a long-haul flight, suspect DVT and calculate Wells score +/– do D-dimer.

Another way to narrow down differentials is by determining which zone the pain predominates (Figure 8.2a and b).

Zone 1: Upper third of posteromedial tibial border to tibial plateau

Zone 2: Middle third of posteromedial tibial border

Zone 3: Distal third of posteromedial tibial border

Zone 4: Anterior tibial border to lateral border of anterior compartment

Zone 5: Inferior patellar margin to tibial tuberosity

Zone 6: Posterior knee skin folds to base of heel and lateral borders of gastrocnemius-solus complex

Zone 1, 2 and 3 ΔΔ: MTSS, stress fracture, muscle injury, tendinopathy, superficial peroneal nerve entrapment or referred

Zone 4 ΔΔ: Anterior CECS, peripheral nerve entrapment, muscle injury, tendinopathy, stress fracture or referred

Zone 5ΔΔ: See Figure 8.1 zone "F" above

Zone 6 ΔΔ: Muscle injury, deep or superficial CECS, PAES, tendinopathy or referred

MEDIAL TIBIAL STRESS SYNDROME (MTSS)

A condition characterised by bony overload, common in runners and military recruits, associated with periostitis, possibly secondary to repetitive muscle traction.

Clinical features:

- Diffuse pain on distal two-thirds of the medial tibial border
- Provoked during or after exercise, can decrease as athlete warms up, but reduces with relative rest
- Scrutinise training history as an aetiological factor

Examination:

- Tenderness on posteromedial tibial border at muscular insertions
- May have tight and weak posterior chain
- Look for predisposing features, e.g. pes planus, poor hip or ankle ROM, increased body mass index (BMI), increased calf girth

Investigations:

- Clinical diagnosis, but imaging can help differentiate other pathology
- Vitamin D

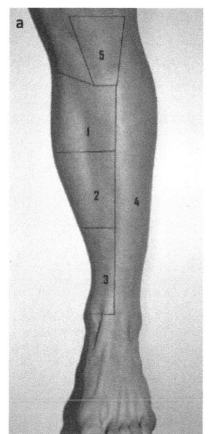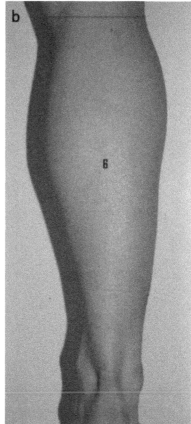

Figure 8.2 (a) Anterior zones for leg pain and (b) posterior zone for leg pain. (Reproduced with kind permission from the Defence Medical Rehabilitation Centre [Stanford Hall].)

- X-ray will normally be negative
- MRI may show diffuse oedema + periosteal thickening

Management:

- Activity modification with relative rest as pain allows
- Graded rehabilitation programme focussed on muscle strength and endurance followed by return to running programme
- Address risk factors: Education regarding training load, biomechanical correction with orthoses or taping, vitamin D supplementation if insufficient
- Gait retraining has proven to be successful in military personnel (2)
- Interventional options may include ESWT

BONE STRESS REACTION/ FRACTURE OF TIBIA OR FIBULA

Clinical features:

- Localised sharp pain on medial tibial surface or fibula (frank fractures may have pain on walking or rest pain)

- Pain worse with impact, e.g. running, jumping
- Scrutinise training history and nutritional/ menstrual history to assess possible underlying aetiology

Examination:

- Pain localised to tibia or fibula
- Hop test +
- Pain when tapping over area (percussion tenderness)
- +/− Pain with tuning fork

Investigations:

- Bloods: Full blood count (FBC), urea and electrolytes (U&Es), liver function tests (LFTs), bone profile, consider phosphate (PO_4^{2-}) and parathyroid hormone (PTH), vitamin D, ferritin and iron studies, thyroid function tests (TFTs) +/− anti-TTG for coeliac screen, sex hormones
- Imaging:
  - X-ray: Can be negative initially, if longstanding may be callous formation or periosteal reaction
  - MRI most sensitive modality – shows periosteal and bone marrow oedema

Table 8.4 Clinical and radiological features of medial tibial stress injuries as per the Fredericson classification and estimated return to play times

Clinical features	Grade	X-ray	MRI	Management/RTP
Post-exercise pain	1	Normal	+ STIR	3 weeks
Pain during exercise	2	Normal	+ STIR and T2WI	3–6 weeks
Pain walking	3	Discrete line or periosteal reaction	+T1WI and T2WI but without cortical break	12–16 weeks
Rest pain	4	Fracture or periosteal reaction	+T1WI and T2WI with fracture line	>16 weeks

STIR, short-tau inversion recovery; T1WI, T1-weighted image; T2WI, T2-weighted image; RTP, return to play.

Fredericson initially described an MRI classification system for medial tibial bone stress which can be useful to prognosticate RTP time (see Table 8.4) (3). There is also the Arendt grading system which incorporates short tau inversion recovery (STIR) (4).

Fredericson classification

Grade 0 – Normal
Grade 1 – Periosteal oedema
Grade 2 – Marrow oedema visible on T2 MRI
Grade 3 – Marrow oedema visible on T1 and T2
Grade 4a – Intracortical signal changes
Grade 4b – Linear region of intracortical signal change

Management of lower limb stress fractures (low risk):

- Offload with activity modification and relative rest +/– crutch if pain on weight bearing
- Analgesia (not non-steroidal anti-inflammatories [NSAIDs] as can impair bony healing)
- Address underlying cause, e.g. education re: training loads, formal biomechanical assessment
- Optimise lifestyle measures, e.g. Stop smoking, dietary advice if under-fuelling and vitamin D supplementation if insufficient or deficient
- Maintain ROM and CV fitness – swim, cycle, upper body strength and trunk stability
- Graded rehabilitation programme
  - Progressive lower limb strengthening programme
  - Increase loading and introduce plyometrics once progressed through strengthening programme without worsening pain
- Return to play governed by clinical assessment of pain, strength and ROM
- Address psychological aspects and involve multidisciplinary team (MDT) if in an elite setting including coach, dietician, psychologist

- If refractory consider novel agents: antiresorptive (bisphosphonates, denosumab) and anabolic (PTH) – may require specialist input, e.g. metabolic bone centre

Management of high-risk tibial stress fractures:

- If involvement of the anterior cortex of the tibia then there is a high risk of non-union. This requires surgical referral for consideration of intramedullary nailing +/– bone graft.
- Period of relative offloading followed by the above management plan.

For a full breakdown of low and high risk stress fractures please see Chapter 12.

CHRONIC EXERTIONAL COMPARTMENT SYNDROME (CECS)

The exact underlying pathophysiology of CECS remains unclear. It is thought to be secondary to fascial non-compliance with sparse evidence for muscle ischaemia. It has also been described as secondary to biomechanical muscle overload in a military population (5).

Clinical features:

- Aching, burning or 'tightness' in legs, commonly bilateral
- Crescendo pain
- Occurs during exertion (normally about 10 minutes into exercise) which is relieved with rest, e.g. running, tabbing, walking fast or uphill
- May be accompanied by paraesthesia and/or numbness of leg and foot on exertion
- Audible "foot slapping" (due to fatigue of tibialis anterior)
- Muscle herniation

Table 8.5 Clinical features of chronic exertional compartment syndrome according to compartment involved

Anterior compartment (most common)	Lateral compartment	Posterior compartment
• Tibialis anterior, EDL, EHL • *Deep peroneal nerve* • Paraesthesia 1st web space • +/− Weak ankle dorsiflexion • May complain of 'foot slapping' when running	• Peroneal longus and brevis • *Superficial peroneal nerve* • Paraesthesia lateral ankle • +/− Weak eversion	• Tib post, FHL, FDL (deep) and gastroc and soleus (superficial) • *Tibial nerve* • Paraesthesia heel of foot • +/− weak plantarflexion

EDL, extensory digitorum lnogus; EHL, extensor hallucis longus; FHL, flexor hallucis longus.

• Clinical features divided by compartment are summarised in Table 8.5

Examination:

• Can have a normal examination
• May have tenderness +/− swelling or muscle herniation in affected compartment after exercise
• Assess for paraesthesia

Pedowitz criteria

Normal: 0–10 mmHg

1 or more of:

Baseline ICP	>15 mmHg
1-min post-exertion	>30 mmHg
5-min post-exertion	>20 mmHg

Investigations:

• X-ray: Negative
• Consider MRI lumbar spine and bilateral lower limbs: Signal hyperintensity on T2WI or STIR
  • Dynamic intra-compartmental pressure (ICP) testing is the gold standard but invasive – Pedowitz criteria (which is performed before and after exercise) or dynamic pressure testing using the Roscoe (6) or Barnes and Allen (7) criteria (see the box titled 'Pedowitz criteria')

Management:

• Conservative management can be tried with varying success: Gait retraining, orthotics, stretching, training load modification, soft tissue therapy and/or avoidance or provoking activities
• Surgical referral for staged compartment fasciotomy or fasciectomy if refractory and severe symptoms

ΔΔ: Accessory soleus

POPLITEAL ARTERY ENTRAPMENT SYNDROME

PAES is characterised by the extrinsic compression of the popliteal artery by surrounding musculotendinous structures; commonly the medial head of gastrocnemius.

Type I–V is described depending on the anatomical type of entrapment.

Clinical features:

• Intermittent claudication pain in calf which relieves on rest; 25–40% bilateral

Examination:

• At rest lower pulses are normal unless severe stenosis or occlusion.
• Ask to do clinically provocative test, e.g. go for run or repeated plantarflexion.
• Ensure no features of acute limb ischaemia secondary to thrombosis (pain, pulseless, pallor, paralysis, paraesthesia, perishing cold)

Investigations:

• X-rays will be negative
• US duplex: Dynamic obstruction of flow within popliteal artery during plantarflexion
• MRI + angiography during provocation, e.g. plantarflexion

Management:

• If functional, i.e. no evidence of anatomical occlusion, consider trial of ultrasound-guided botulinum toxin A (Botox™) injection at site of occlusion, i.e. medial head of gastrocnemius.
• If symptoms do not resolve or are refractory to Botox, consider surgical referral for musculotendinous release of the popliteal artery.

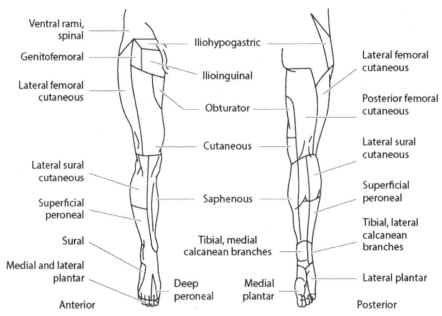

Figure 8.3 Peripheral nerve sensory distribution of the lower leg. (Original image from *Anatomy*, 5th edition, edited by R O'Rahilly. Philadelphia, WB Saunders Company, 1986.)

PERIPHERAL NERVE ENTRAPMENTS

Peripheral nerve innvervation of the lower limbs is summarised in Figure 8.3.

Superficial peroneal nerve entrapment

This is a possible complication following a lateral ankle sprain. Entrapment occurs as the nerve exits the lateral compartment approximately 10cm proximal to the ankle joint.

Clinical features:

- Neuropathic aching pain in the lateral distal calf, often poorly localised
- Worse during or after running
- +/− numbness/paraesthesia over dorsum of foot and lateral ankle
- More common in those with a history of T2DM or thyroid disease

Examination:

- Palpate the common peroneal nerve around head of fibula
- Tinel's test +
- May be an evident fascial defect 10 cm above the lateral malleolus

Investigations: Nerve conduction studies, ultrasound or MRI to assess soft tissue

Management: Mobilisation or surgical referral if refractory symptoms for nerve exploration and release

Deep peroneal nerve

This is a possible complication following lateral ankle sprain. A frequent site of entrapment is behind the inferior extensor retinaculum in the 'anterior tarsal tunnel.'

Clinical features: Pain or paraesthesia dorsum of foot which can radiate to the 1st web space

Examination:

- Palpate common peroneal nerve around head of fibula
- Tinel's test +
- Plantarflexion worsens symptoms (stretches nerve)

Investigations: Nerve conduction studies, X-ray to assess for bony abnormalities, e.g. osteophytes, MRI to assess soft tissue

Management: Conservative including shoe alterations or physiotherapy if ankle instability. Consider surgical referral for decompression if refractory

Sural nerve entrapment

The sural nerve is a pure sensory nerve formed by terminal branches of the tibial and common peroneal nerves.

Common causes of damage or entrapment include:

- Trauma
- Fracture of the calcaneus
- Iatrogenic, e.g. post-surgery

Clinical features: Entrapment causes paraesthesia in the lower lateral leg, lateral heel and foot

CALF MUSCLE INJURY

Injury to the medial gastrocnemius (most common), soleus or plantaris.

Mechanism of injury: Forceful contraction of calf or acceleration, e.g. jumping, sprinting or eccentric overstretch

Clinical features:

- Calf pain
- Swelling or ecchymosis
- Loss of function
- May report a sudden 'pop' felt in calf

Examination:

- Antalgic gait
- Tenderness to palpation over affected muscle
- Swelling and/or ecchymosis
- Pain on resisted plantarflexion or passive stretch
- Perform Simmond's test to rule out Achilles tendon rupture

Investigations: US to characterise muscle, musculo-tendinous junction (MTJ) or tendinous involvement

Classification by Pedret (8) characterised five injury types according to characteristics. The worst prognoses were injuries associated with the free aponeurosis (types 3 and 4).

Management for medial gastrocnemius muscle injury:

Acute phase
- Protect, ice, optimal loading, compression, elevation (POLICE), analgesia
- Muscle activation 3–4×/day, low-grade pain free, e.g. plantarflexion with foot against wall whilst lying supine
- Aim for pain-free walking and restore ROM
- Maintain CV fitness throughout, e.g. rowing, stationary cycle, stepper

Can progress to the next stage when walking pain free and isometrics can be performed pain free.

Subacute phase:
1. Muscle strengthening
   - Muscle strengthening of gastrocnemius and soleus, 3 sets of 12 repetitions:
     - E.g. heel raises, initially double, then progress to single. Also perform with bent knee to isolate soleus.
     - TheraBand™ exercises

- Delay eccentric exercises until later in rehabilitation, especially if tendon involvement
- Muscle strengthening of kinetic chain
  - Squats, deep lunge, hamstring curls
- Neuromuscular (NM) control - proprioceptive exercises on BOSU

Progress when can perform the above pain free, with good form and no guarding.

2. Functional exercises
   - Return to running programme
   - Sport-specific drills, e.g. fast feet

3. Maintain CV fitness throughout
4. Attend training and address risk factors, e.g. muscle weakness or imbalances

Progress to training when minimal symptoms and a return to running programme has been completed, there is full and pain-free ROM.

Return to play: Return to play once completed one week of full training

REFERENCES

1. Sihvonen R, Paavola M, Malmivaara A, Itälä A, Joukainen A, Nurmi H, et al. Arthroscopic partial meniscectomy versus sham surgery for a degenerative meniscal tear. *New Eng J Med.* 2013;369(26): 2515–24.
2. Sharma J, Weston M, Batterham AM, Spears IR. Gait retraining and incidence of medial tibial stress syndrome in army recruits. *Med Sci Sports Exerc.* 2014;46(9): 1684–92.
3. Fredericson M, Bergman AG, Hoffman KL, Dillingham MS. Tibial stress reaction in runners. Correlation of clinical symptoms and scintigraphy with a new magnetic resonance imaging grading system. *Am J Sports Med.* 1995;23(4):472–81.
4. Arendt E, Agel J, Heikes C, Griffiths H. Stress injuries to bone in college athletes: A retrospective review of experience at a single institution. *Am J Sports Med.* 2003;31(6):959–68.
5. Franklyn-Miller A, Roberts A, Hulse D, Foster J. Biomechanical overload syndrome: Defining a new diagnosis. *Br J Sports Med.* 2014;48(6):415–6.
6. Pedowitz RA, Hargens AR, Mubarak SJ, Gershuni DH. Modified criteria for the objective diagnosis of chronic compartment syndrome of the leg. *Am J Sports Med.* 1990;18(1):35–40.
7. Allen M, Barnes M. Exercise pain in the lower leg. Chronic compartment syndrome and medial tibial syndrome. *J Bone Joint Surg Br.* 1986;68:818–23.
8. Pedret C, Balius R, Blasi M, Dávila F, Aramendi JF, Masci L, et al. Ultrasound classification of medial gastrocnemious injuries. *Scand J Med Sci Sports.* 2020;30(12):2456–65.

9 Foot and ankle

ACHILLES TENDON

"This 32-year-old amateur runner has presented to a general sports medicine clinic with an insidious onset of posterior foot/heel pain and swelling. They are currently training for their first marathon which is in 4 months. Please take and history and do a focussed examination and discuss a management plan."

Differential diagnoses:

- Midportion tendon pathology – tendinopathy, partial tear, full rupture
- Insertional tendon pathology – tendinopathy, retrocalcaneal bursitis
- Posterior ankle impingement
- Flexor hallucis longus (FHL) or tibialis posterior tendinopathy
- Sever's disease
- Spondyloarthropathy (SpA)
- Calcaneal stress fracture
- Referred pain from spine

ACHILLES TENDINOPATHY

Midportion Achilles tendinopathy

Risk factors for midportion Achilles tendinopathy are summarised in Table 9.1.

Clinical features:

- Pain after exercise +/– first thing in the morning
- Pain at start of activity but then 'warms up'
- Associated with a recent change in load and/ or metabolic abnormality
- Ask about rheumatological symptoms, medications and family history

Examination:

- Local tenderness and possible thickening of the tendon
- Frank swelling and crepitus may indicate a tenosynovitis
- Assess for manifestations of seronegative arthropathy, e.g. restricted lumbar spine range of movement (ROM), uveitis, psoriasis

Investigations:

- Not always necessary
- Assess for risk factors: Blood sugar (BM), fasting blood glucose, urea and electrolytes (U&E), lipids, possible rheumatological screen, e.g. C-reactive protein (CRP), erythrocyte sedimentation rate (ESR), HLA B27
- Ultrasound (US): Hypo-echogenicity, thickened tendon, neovascularisation
- X-ray: To assess for differentials
- Magnetic resonance imaging (MRI) if refractory or diagnosis unclear (see Chapter 18)

Management:

- Education on pathology and treatment
  - Activity modification and relative load reduction
  - Analgesia including ice and paracetamol
  - Rehabilitation course average 3–6 months and 10–50% do not respond
  - Expect noticeable change in symptoms by 4 weeks
- Educate on training loads and vary training programme
- Address any risk factors, e.g. poorly controlled diabetes, dietary input if obese
- Rehabilitation
  - Isometric exercises – 45 seconds holding a calf raise, five repetitions (perform seated if significant pain) with body weight or free weights

Progress once pain <5/10, no morning stiffness, low pain on single leg calf raise

- Isotonic exercises (continue isometrics alongside)
  - Slow and heavy concentric and eccentric, e.g. calf raises 3 seconds up and 4 seconds down, three sets of eight repetitions on alternate days (or 3×/week)
  - Strengthen soleus and kinetic chain, e.g. quadriceps and gluteals
  - Avoid loading on consecutive days, at least initially

DOI: 10.1201/9781003163701-11

Table 9.1 Intrinsic and extrinsic risk factors predisposing to midportion Achilles tendinopathy

Intrinsic risk factors	Extrinsic risk factors
Obesity and metabolic syndrome	Change in loading
Renal failure	• Distance, frequency, recovery
Inflammatory arthritis	Change in surface
Hypercholesterolaemia	Change in footwear
Genetic	Poor technique
Medications – steroids/ fluoroquinolones	
Pes cavus	
Lateral ankle instability	
Muscle imbalance or weakness	

- Energy storage (Continue isotonics twice per week)
  - Twice per week, e.g. double leg hop, forward and backwards hop, side to side then single leg hop
- Sport specific, e.g. return to running programme, jumping, ball drills, change of direction

RTP when can do above without exacerbation of pain

- Other – podiatry input or manual therapy to trigger points in muscles
- Refractory cases – consider dry needling, glceryl trinitrate (GTN), sclerosing therapies. Studies have shown steroid injections have no long-term benefit and are associated with a risk of tendon rupture (1, 2)
- Adjuncts include extra corporal shock wave therapy (ESWT)
- Surgery is generally considered as a last resort. Currently there is no randomised controlled trial (RCT) comparing surgical vs conservative management

Insertional tendinopathy

Insertional tendinopathy encompasses tendinopathy of the Achilles tendon insertion, retrocalcaneal bursitis and Achilles bursitis.

If features are bilateral, then assess for other features of SpA.

Management has the same principles as midportion tendinopathy as above, however rehabilitation should avoid dorsiflexion which compresses local structures and consider the use of a heel raise. Bursitis may benefit from a steroid injection. In refractory cases consider ESWT, autologous blood injection (ABI) or surgery.

ΔΔ: SpA, gout, drug mediated (fluoroquinolones, e.g. ciprofloxacin), metabolic, e.g. type II diabetes mellitus (T2DM), plantaris tendon (medial)

Posterior ankle impingement

Impingement of the posterior talus by the posterior tibia, typically in plantarflexion, e.g. ballet, pushing off.

Predisposing factors:

- Os trigonum
- Enlarged posterior tubercle of talus (Stieda process)
- Lateral talar process fracture

Clinical features: Pain deep to the Achilles tendon

Examination:

- Posterior impingement + (passive overpressure with plantarflexion)
- Assess Flexor Hallucis Longus (FHL), as commonly pathology coexists

Investigations:

- X-rays (anteroposterior [AP] and lateral views) can assess for an Os trigonum or other osseous abnormalities
- MRI: Localised fluid, accompanying bone contusion, posterolateral capsular thickening and synovitis

Management:

Conservative:
- Modify activities – reduce extreme plantarflexion
- Analgesia
- Manual mobilisation if stiff subtalar or talocrural joint
- Muscle strengthening programme for plantarflexors
- Taping to reduce end ROM plantarflexion

Surgical referral if symptoms refractory to conservative treatment, e.g. excision of os trigonum.

Achilles tendon rupture

Mechanism of injury (MOI): Sudden planter flexion, common in middle aged men.

Predisposing factors include previous intratendon steroid injection, T2DM, gout, fluoroquinolone antibiotics, hyperparathyroidism and rheumatoid arthritis.

Clinical features:

- Sudden pain in heel,
- May report a 'pop' in the back of the leg or that someone has kicked them
- Loss of function

Examination:

- Palpable defect in the tendon
- Loss of normal planter-flexed resting position of foot
- Weak plantar flexion
- Simmond's test+

Investigations:

- X-rays: Soft tissue swelling and obliteration of the pre-Achilles fat pad (Kager's triangle)
- US or MRI can demonstrate the degree of tear

Management:

- Equinus boot for 2 weeks, then change boot and early mobilisation followed by progressive rehabilitation programme. A recent RCT showed no benefit of surgery vs conservative management (3)

ANKLE PAIN

Common causes of ankle pain are summarised in Table 9.2.

ACUTE INJURIES

Lateral ankle ligament injury

Mechanism of injury: Commonly after an inversion injury.

Ligaments involved include the anterior talofibular ligament (ATFL), the calcaneofibular ligament (CFL) and the posterior talofibular ligament (PTFL) (Figure 9.1).

Injuries to the ATFL are most common (ATFL > CFL > PTFL).

Clinical features:

- Lateral ankle pain,
- Swelling or ecchymosis,
- Instability

Examination:

- Antalgic gait, swelling and bruising around anterior and lateral joint line, tender palpating affected ligament +/– lateral malleolus
- Pain on plantarflexion/inversion, in more severe cases eversion may be weak due to peroneal nerve traction injury
- Anterior drawer +, squeeze + and external rotation (ER) + if syndesmosis involved

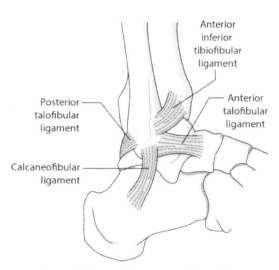

Figure 9.1 Lateral ligaments of the ankle. (Reproduced with kind permission from *Orthopaedic Trauma: The Stanmore and Royal London Guide*, CRC Press, 2015.)

Investigations:

- X-ray (AP, lateral and mortise views) if Ottowa rules + or suspect syndesmosis injury (see the box titled 'Ottowa ankle rules')
- US or MRI if refractory pain. MRI may show discontinuity of the ligament, detachment, contour irregularity or possibly intrasubstance oedema (see Chapter 18)

Ottowa ankle rules

- Bony tenderness medial or lateral malleolus,
- Bony tenderness navicular or base of 5th metatarsal
- Unable to weight bear four steps

Syndesmosis injury:

- Tibfib overlap should be >6 mm on AP or >1 mm on mortise view with medial clear space <4 mm

---

Table 9.2 Differential diagnosis of ankle pain according to location

Medial ankle pain	Anterior ankle pain	Lateral ankle pain
Tibialis posterior tendinopathy	Tibialis anterior tendinopathy	Peroneal tendinopathy
FHL tendinopathy	Sinus tarsi syndrome	Sinus tarsi syndrome
Tarsal tunnel syndrome	Anterior impingement	Stress fracture talus or fibula
Posterior impingement	Superficial peroneal nerve entrapment	Referred: Lumbar spine
Navicular stress fracture		Sural nerve entrapment
Referred: Lumbar spine L4		
FHL, flexor hallucis longus.		

Management:

Acute phase:
- Activity modification +/– crutch if painful to walk
- Protect, optimal loading, ice, compression, elevation (POLICE)
- Gradual WB to restore normal gait
- Analgesia (not non-steroidal anti-inflammatories [NSAIDs] for first 72 hours)
- Gentle active range of movement (ROM) exercises, e.g. write alphabet with ankle

Subacute phase:
- Muscle conditioning – TheraBand™ eversion and dorsiflexion, heel raises
- ROM – Knee to wall exercises
- Proprioception – single leg standing with eyes closed, then progress to wobble board exercises
- Continue cardiovascular (CV) fitness, e.g. stationary cycling

Return to play (RTP):
- Return to running
- Add dynamic movement
- Sport-specific training
- RTP once one-week full training and functional exercises do not provoke pain
- Some find taping can initially be beneficial

If a patient presents with refractory symptoms despite full rehabilitation programme, consider other injuries complicating lateral ankle sprain, such as:

- Talar dome pathology, e.g. osteochondral lesion – especially if there was a compressive element to the MOI
- Syndesmosis injury +/– Maisonneuve (remember to palpate the entire fibula)
- Tarsal coalition
- Sinus tarsi – may require further investigation such as MRI
- Chronic instability is common and may require an ongoing proprioception and strengthening programme to prevent re-injury

Fifth metatarsal (MT) fractures

Fifth MT fractures can be subsequent to direct trauma, crushing or twisting. The different zones of injury are represented in Figure 9.2.

Zone 1: Avulsion – tuberosity
- An avulsion fracture (transverse or oblique) of the tuberosity which often accompanies inversion ankle injury at the site of insertion of peroneus brevis
- Plantarflexion and inversion

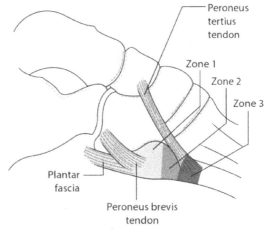

Figure 9.2 The zones of the proximal fifth metatarsal and their anatomical relations. (Reproduced with kind permission from *Orthopaedic Trauma: The Stanmore and Royal London Guide*, CRC Press, 2015.)

- Management: Conservative with boot/stiff shoe, weight-bear (WB) as tolerated
Zone 2: Jones fracture – metaphyseal-diaphyseal junction (within 1.5 cm of tuberosity)
- A Jones fracture is a horizontal fracture that extends into the intertarsal joint of the 4th–5th articulation, commonly in athletes
- Vascular watershed area – high risk of non-union
- Management: Orthopaedic referral for possible screw fixation. Short leg cast with non-weight bearing (NWB) for 6 weeks
Zone 3: Stress fracture – diaphysis
- Stress fracture of proximal diaphysis, distal to the 4th–5th MT articulation
- High risk of non-union
- Management: Orthopaedic referral with NWB short leg cast for 6 weeks

Investigations: AP, lateral and oblique X-ray views according to Ottowa rules

Ensure you don't miss Lisfranc injuries with 5th MT fractures.

MEDIAL ANKLE PAIN
Tibialis posterior tendinopathy

Mechanism of injury: Overuse injury of the primary evertor of the foot. Associated with rear foot valgus

Clinical features:

- Medial ankle pain posterior to medial malleolus which can extend to its insertion on the navicular
- Pain on resisted inversion and passive eversion

NORMAL FOOT

TARSAL TUNNEL SYNDROME

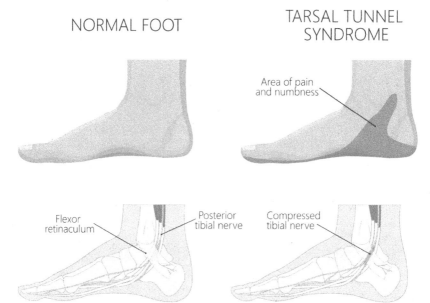

Figure 9.3 Distribution of symptoms in tarsal tunnel syndrome.

Investigations: US or MRI

Management:

- Activity modification and analgesia
- Orthotics if excessive pronation
- Graduated strengthening programme especially inversion and plantar flexion

Flexor hallucis longus (FHL) tendinopathy

Overuse injury of FHL associated with plantarflexion and ballet 'en pointe'.

Clinical features:

- Pain in posterior ankle or plantar surface of great toe associated with plantarflexion or when pointing toes +/− crepitus

Examination:

- Pain on resisted flexion of hallux or passive extension
- If severe, may cause triggering of hallux

Investigations: US or MRI

Management:

- Activity modification and analgesia
- Technique adjustment
- Orthotics if excessive pronation
- Graduated strengthening programme focussing on FHL

ΔΔ: Sesamoiditis or sesamoid stress fracture.

Tarsal tunnel syndrome

Entrapment of the posterior tibial nerve within the tarsal tunnel behind the medial malleolus.

It can be idiopathic or secondary to injury, pronation, footwear or occasionally from an osseous structure, e.g. osteophytes.

Clinical features:

- Vague medial ankle "burning pain" which can radiate to the arch of the foot (Figure 9.3)
- +/− Paraesthesia
- Exacerbated by prolonged standing or walking

Examination: Tinel's test +, local tenderness, pes planus

Investigations:

- It is a clinical diagnosis
- X-ray and MRI can delineate bony and soft tissue surrounding structures
- Electromyography (EMG) can help confirm the diagnosis

Management:

- Activity modification
- Analgesia
- Orthotic referral
- Surgical release

LATERAL ANKLE PAIN

Peroneal tendinopathy

Mechanism of injury: Overuse injury commonly of peroneus brevis

Clinical features:

- Pain behind lateral malleolus extending to base of 5th MT
- +/− retromalleolar swelling

Examination:

- Local tenderness +/− swelling and crepitus
- Painful resisted eversion
- Calf tightness
- Stiff subtalar joint

Investigations: US or MRI

Management:

- Activity modification and analgesia
- Mobilise subtalar joint
- Strengthening programme focussing on eversion
- Biomechanical and footwear assessment

Sinus tarsi syndrome

Inflammation of the small osseous canal between the talus and calcaneum. It is common after lateral ankle injury.

Clinical features:

- Vague lateral/anterior ankle pain,
- Pain when on uneven surfaces

Examination:

- Stiff subtalar joint
- Pain on end range inversion or eversion

Investigations: Diagnostic local anaesthetic (LA) injection, X-ray and/or MRI

Management:

- Manual therapy to mobilise subtalar joint
- Correction of predisposing biomechanical abnormalities
- Therapeutic corticosteroid injection
- Surgical options for excision of inflammatory tissue/cyst if present

ANTERIOR ANKLE PAIN

Tibialis anterior tendinopathy

This is an overuse injury of tibialis anterior which is the primary dorsiflexor of foot. It's origin is the lateral shaft and condyle of the tibia and its insertion is middle cuneiform and base of the 1st MT. It is common from hill running or tight boots.

Clinical features: Pain and swelling over the anterior ankle, worse with activity

Examination: Pain on resisted dorsiflexion

Investigations: US or MRI

Management:

- Activity modification
- Analgesia
- Training load education
- Correct biomechanics, e.g. orthotics or reducing stride length
- Strengthening programme

Anterior ankle impingement

Compression of soft tissue or osseous structures at the anterior margin of the tibiotalar joint during dorsiflexion, e.g. osteophytes or exotoses. It is common in football and ballet.

Clinical features: Pain in anterior ankle during dorsiflexion

Examination:

- Tenderness on palpation of the anterior joint line
- Painful and restricted ROM in dorsiflexion
- Anterior impingement +

Investigations:

- X-ray: Lateral ankle X-ray will show bony exostoses at the anterior tibial margin (see Chapter 18)
- US/MRI

Management:

- Activity modification +/− heel lift
- Analgesia, e.g. NSAIDs
- Taping to reduce end ROM
- Strengthening programme
- Surgical removal of exotoses

FOOT PAIN

Plantar fasciitis

Inflammation of the plantar fasciia at the medial process of the calcaneal tuberosity secondary to repetitive traction. It is common in patients with a high BMI and pes planus or poorly fitting footwear.

Clinical features: Gradual onset pain medial aspect of heel worse in the morning

Examination: Pinpoint tenderness at the medial process of the calcaneal tuberosity, pain on hallux dorsiflexion

Investigations:

- It is a clinical diagnosis
- X-ray or MRI can help assess for calcaneal stress fracture as differential
- US can assess for a partial tear which may limit possible adjunctive treatment options.

Management:

- Activity modification and analgesia
- Education regarding training loads
- Correct biomechanical abnormalities, e.g. orthoses, taping
- Stretching
- Strengthening programme – e.g. heel raises with towel under hallux, calf strengthening and proximal kinetic chain
- Referral to dietician if overweight
- Consider night splint or Strasbourg sock for refractory pain
- Consider corticosteroid injection, ABI or ESWT (evidence inconclusive)

ΔΔ: Calcaneal stress fracture, medial plantar nerve entrapment.

Navicular stress fracture

Mechanism of injury: Overuse injury associated with reduced ankle dorsiflexion. It is a high risk injury (high risk of avascular necrosis [AVN]) due to avascularity of the central third of the navicular bone.

Clinical features: Midfoot pain +/− swelling, pain on loading

Examination: Tender to direct palpation of the navicular and/or midfoot

Investigations: X-ray may miss early change, MRI shows high signal on T2WI

Management:

- Cast immobilisation for 6–8 weeks followed by progression rehabilitation programme
- Surgical open reduction internal fixation (ORIF) if failed conservative management or non-union and consideration in elite athletes

ΔΔ: Os naviculare, tibialis posterior tendinopathy.

Tarsal coalition

Tarsal coalition refers to a group of conditions where there is a complete or partial union between two or three tarsal bones. Fusion can either be (a) osseous (b) cartilaginous or (c) fibrous. The most common coalitions are:

- Calcaneonavicular
- Talocalcaneal
- Calcaneocuboid

Clinical features:

- Asymptomatic
- Midfoot or hindfoot pain or stiffness

- May present with 'recurrent ankle sprains'
- Rigid pes planus
- Limited subtalar ROM

Investigations:

- X-ray: Normally first line and should include AP, standing lateral, Harris views (axial calcaneal projection) and 45° internal oblique view
  - Calcaneonavicular coalition may be demonstrated with an 'anteater sign' (see Chapter 18) which refers to an anterior elongation of the superior calcaneus which overlaps the navicular on lateral X-ray
  - Talocalcaneal coalition may be demonstrated on lateral X-ray with a talar beak or characteristic 'c-sign' which is an arc formed by the medial outline of the talar dome and posteroinferior aspect of sustentaculum tali
- Computed tomography (CT) can help to determine the size and location of the coalition whilst MRI is useful to visualise cartilaginous or fibrous bridges

Management:

- Conservative management includes activity modification, orthotics and NSAIDs. Below knee casting can also be used temporarily in severe cases.
- Surgical treatment can be offered in refractory cases and options include (a) coalition resection, (b) subtalar fusion or c) triple fusion.

GREAT TOE

Sesamoid pathology

"An elite shot putter presents with a 4-month history of pain under her great toe, worse when she pushes off with her right foot."

Mechanism of injury: forced dorsiflexion of the first metatarsophalangeal (MTP) joint, e.g. ballet, sprint start. The medial sesamoid is the most commonly affected.

Clinical features: Hallux pain, especially on loading or toe-off phase of gait, swelling

Examination:

- Tendency to supinate foot during gait to reduce pressure on sesamoid
- Tenderness to direct palpation

- Restricted ROM of hallux
- Pain on resisted hallux plantarflexion

Investigations:

- X-rays (AP and lateral foot, medical oblique and axial sesamoid view)
- MRI: Bone marrow oedema if inflammation

Management:

- Conservative management: padding, taping and orthotics with activity modification
- In sesamoiditis consider US-guided injection of steroid + LA
- Sesamoidectomy if refractory

ΔΔ: Sesamoiditis, stress fracture, sprain 'turf toe', FHL or FHL tendinopathy, osteoarthritis (OA).

REFERENCES

1. Coombes BK, Bisset L, Vicenzino B. Efficacy and safety of corticosteroid injections and other injections for management of tendinopathy: A systematic review of randomised controlled trials. *Lancet.* 2010;376:1751–67.
2. Kearney RS, Parsons N, Metcalfe D, Costa ML. Injection therapies for Achilles tendinopathy. *Cochrane Database Syst Rev.* 2015(5):CD010960.
3. Maempel JF, Clement ND, Wickramasinghe NR, Duckworth AD, Keating JF. Operative repair of acute Achilles tendon rupture does not give superior patient-reported outcomes to nonoperative management. *Bone Joint J.* 2020;102-B(7):933–40.

SPECIAL GROUPS

PAEDIATRIC PRESENTATIONS

Paediatric cases have come up in previous objective structured clinical examinations (OSCEs) and have included some of the common paediatric musculoskeletal pathology listed below, as well as concussion (see Chapter 13). Stations have almost always also included parents present, and often there is a strong emphasis on communication as well as achieving the correct clinical diagnosis. Red flag symptoms should always be explored such as systemic upset or signs of malignancy. Consider the child's developmental age, and how this may affect the prognosis and management of their injury, i.e. if there is still a significant amount of growth expected. In addition, explore the wider community around the patient, e.g. school, peers, sports teams and whether there is an underlying safeguarding issue that may be feeding into their presentation that you should address.

Long bone anatomy in paediatrics differs to that in adults (see Figure 10.1). In paediatric long bones, as well as the diaphysis and the metaphysis there is also the physis/epiphyseal growth plate and the epiphysis which is the rounded end of a long bone that is part of the joint. In addition, paediatric patients have apophyses which are normal bony outgrowths with a musculotendinous unit attached to it. This eventually fuses over time. The difference in this anatomy leads to different patterns of injuries in paediatric populations compared with adults.

Special considerations in paediatrics:

- Developmental age
- Growth plate injuries
- Safeguarding

OSGOOD-SCHLATTER DISEASE

"You have been referred a 12-year-old school child by his General Practitioner (GP) for persistent knee pain. He currently plays hockey, football and cricket for the school and county rugby and football. His symptoms are specifically at the tibial tuberosity."

Osgood-Schlatter disease is a type of traction apophysitis (nonarticular osteochondrosis) which describes a group of conditions affecting the immature skeleton. Apophyses are bony outgrowths that arise from separate ossification centres which later fuse and are the site of a tendon or ligament attachment. Commonly encountered conditions include:

- Osgood-Schlatter disease – tibial tuberosity
- Sinding-Larssen-Johannsen disease – inferior patellar pole
- Sever's disease – calcaneus
- Iselin's disease – fifth metatarsal head

Age of onset 12–15 years in males, 8–12 years in females –M:F 4:1

Clinical features:

- Insidious onset of pain and swelling over tibial tubercle
- Symptoms exacerbated during periods of growth and by jumping and running

Examination:

- Point tenderness and bony swelling over the tibial tubercle
- Quadriceps tightness (restricted knee flexion)
- Pain on resisted knee extension
- May have biomechanical abnormalities, e.g. pes planus
- May have patellofemoral (PFP) problems if prolonged

DOI: 10.1201/9781003163701-12

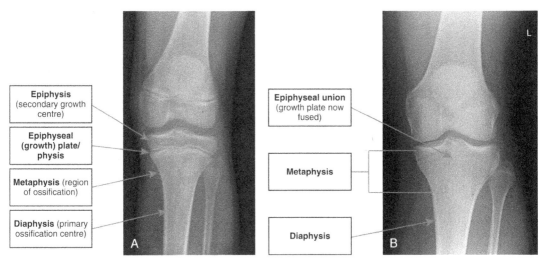

Figure 10.1 Radiological differences of (A) a paediatric left knee and (B) an adult left knee demonstrated on X-ray. (This figure was published in a *Comprehensive Guide to Sports Physiology and Injury Management*, Porter and Wilson, page 380, Copyright Elsevier, 2021.)

Investigations:

- This is normally a clinical diagnosis.
- X-ray if diagnosis is in doubt or persistent symptoms – may show calcification or to rule out avulsion fracture
- Ultrasound (US): To assess for patellar tendinopathy as a differential

If bilateral Sever's consider workup for spondyloarthropathy (SpA)

Management: (Use the same approach for other traction apophysitis)

- Education
  - Explain that likely to last several seasons and symptoms will be worse during periods of rapid growth
  - Excellent prognosis: 95% self-limit
- Activity modification – common in children who do multiple sports frequently. Come to a shared decision with patient and family to potentially cut down the number of aggravating activities and focus on a few favoured sports
  - Involve school coaches and parents so everyone on board, e.g. provide a written letter
- Analgesia – can include topical non-steroidal anti-inflammatories (NSAIDs) and ice over area after sport and to limit oral NSAIDs for important training sessions or big competitions to reduce side effects
- Quadriceps flexibility and strengthening programme — to reduce traction of tight muscle on tibial tuberosity
  - E.g. Shoulder bridges, squats
  - Quadriceps stretches

- Correct any biomechanical abnormalities – check footwear including school shoes
- Consider further imaging and surgical review if skeletally mature and persistent and disabling symptoms

PROXIMAL HUMERAL EPIPHYSIOLITIS

This is caused by repetitive microtrauma to the immature skeleton. It is regarded as a Salter-Harris type I stress injury to proximal humeral physis (see Figure 10.2 and the box titled 'Salter-Harris classification of physeal fractures' for classification).

Common in overhead athletes age 11–16 years.

Salter-Harris classification of physeal fractures

I	Slipped
II	Above physis
III	Lower than physis
IV	Through Everything
V	Rammed

Clinical features: Diffuse arm pain on throwing which resolves with rest

Examination:

- Often nil
- Can get point tenderness over lateral proximal humerus
- Glenohumeral internal rotation deficit (GIRD)

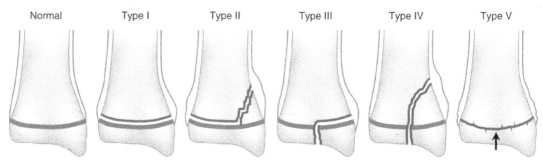

Figure 10.2 Salter-Harris classification of physeal injuries. (This figure was published in *A Comprehensive Guide to Sports Physiology and Injury Management*, Porter and Wilson, page 381, Copyright Elsevier, 2021.)

Investigations:

- X-ray (anteroposterior [AP] in external rotation [ER], scapular y and axillary views) – can be normal. Can get widening of proximal humeral physis (see Chapter 18)
- Magnetic resonance imaging (MRI) – oedema around physis

Management:

- Education – educate patient, coach and parents that pathology is correlated with the number of throws/pitches and mainstay of management is to reduce the number of throws per season to reduce possible complications of growth arrest
- Cessation/reduction of throwing – for at least 2–3 months initially
- Patient can continue to attend training for psychological and team support
- Muscle strengthening programme
  - Rotator cuff (RC) strengthening
  - Posterior shoulder capsule strengthening if GIRD
  - "Thrower's 10" programme
- Prevention
  - Review of technique – avoid late cocking
  - Enforced limits of throwing/pitching
  - Monitor growth and skeletal maturity

AVULSION INJURIES

Apophyseal avulsions occur secondary to a sudden contraction of the muscle at the apophysis. The greatest risk is when muscle strength increases in young athletes with an otherwise immature physis.

Common locations are summarised in Figure 10.3 and include:

Tibial tubercle: Quadriceps
Ischial tuberosity: Hamstrings and/or adductors
Anterior inferior iliac spine (AIIS): Rectus femoris

Anterior superior iliac spine (ASIS): Sartorius or tensor fascia lata
Lesser trochanter: Iliopsoas
Iliac crest: Abdominal muscles

Clinical features:

- Acute 'pop'
- Tenderness to bony origin and muscle involved
- Weakness of muscle involved

Examination:

- Tenderness to palpation over bony insertion and/or muscle
- Weakness and reduced range of movement (ROM)

Investigations:

- X-ray, computed tomography (CT) or MRI

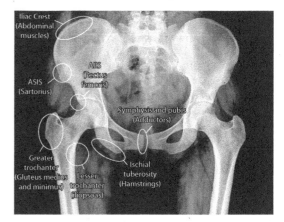

Figure 10.3 AP pelvic X-ray showing the most common locations for paediatric avulsion fractures of the pelvis.

Management:

- In the vast majority management is conservative - treatment as with a high-grade muscle injury
- Surgical referral if a large displacement (exact measurement dependent on location, e.g. >2 cm for ischial tuberosity)

SLIPPED UPPER FEMORAL EPIPHYSIS (SUFE)

Commonly seen in adolescent obese males aged 10–15 years characterised by a slip of the proximal femoral physis. It is generally regarded as a type of Salter-Harris type I injury.

Clinical features:

- Groin, thigh or knee pain +/− limp, which can present acutely or more insidiously over weeks to months
- Approximately 25% are bilateral

Examination:

- High body mass index (BMI)
- Antalgic or waddling gait
- Externally rotated and shortened hip
- Loss of ROM of the hip
- Drehman's sign – passive hip flexion causes external rotation and abduction of the hip which is pathognomonic

Investigations:

- X-ray (AP and frog lateral views) of both hips: Epiphysiolitis, frank slip, measure on AP pelvis using Klein's line (see Chapter 18). Subtle slips may be suggested by a reduction in the height of the physis compared with the contralateral side
- MRI if there is a high clinical suspicion but X-rays are negative

Management:

- Place in wheelchair and urgently refer to orthopaedics for percutaneous pinning
- Discussion regarding lifestyle modification

Possible complications: Osteonecrosis, limb length discrepancy, osteoarthritis.

ADOLESCENT IDIOPATHIC SCOLIOSIS

"A 13-year-old girl presents with thoracic back pain and a complaint of her ribs 'sticking out' on one side which she is becoming increasingly embarrassed about. She has no history of developmental abnormalities. Please take and history and examine this patient."

Adolescent idiopathic scoliosis occurs in an otherwise healthy individual if present after age 10 years. Higher curve angles are more common in females and it is common to have positive family history. It is important to differentiate a structural from a postural scoliosis of which the latter is compensatory to some conditions out with the spine, e.g. short leg or pelvic tilt.

Clinical features:

- Right thoracic curves are most common
- Patients may complain of rib cage protrusion, uneven shoulders, one hip sticking out and/or pain
- Ascertain relevant birth history and if any history of developmental abnormalities
- Ask about height of parents to determine possible remaining growth left

Examination:

- Evaluate body asymmetry: Leg length discrepancy, shoulder height difference, truncal shift (Figure 10.4a)
- Differentiate from postural scoliosis caused by leg length discrepancy by asking patient to sit; the curve should disappear if postural
- Evaluate pubertal development, e.g. Tanner staging
- Neurological examination
- Cutaneous examination for associated conditions, e.g.
  - Café au lait spots and axillary freckles: Neurofibromatosis
  - Hair patch in lumbosacral area: Spina bifida
  - Skin/joint laxity: Marfan's or other connective tissue disorder
- Special tests: Adam's forward bend test will demonstrate rotational element, rib prominence on forward bend test

Investigations:

- X-rays: Spine standing posteroanterior (PA) and lateral views
  - Cobb angle on coronal plane (measurement of lateral spinal curvature) >10° (Figures 10.4b and c).
  - Skeletal maturity can be assessed using the Risser sign on pelvic X-ray (Figure 10.4d). This is important to determine because the curve often progresses during the period of rapid skeletal growth and maturation.

Management:

- Depends on (a) skeletal maturity (can use Tanner or Risser staging and age of menstruation to estimate), (b) severity of scoliosis and (c) progression

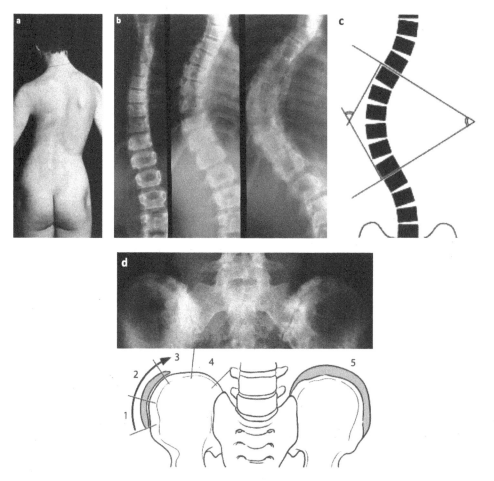

Figure 10.4 Adolescent idiopathic scoliosis: (a) typical thoracic deformity. (b) Serial X-rays showing increased spinal curvature over 4 years. (c) The angle of curvature is measured by Cobb's method: Lines projected from the top of the uppermost and the bottom of the lowermost vertebral bodies in the primary curve define Cobb's angle. (d) Risser's sign: The iliac apophyses normally appear progressively from lateral to medial (stages 1–4). When fusion is complete, spinal maturity has been reached and further increase of curvature is negligible (stage 5). (Reproduced with kind permission from *Apley & Solomon's System of Orthopaedics and Trauma*, 10th edition, CRC Press, 2018.)

- Management can be observation, bracing or surgical
- Regular monitoring if Cobb angle <25°, or <50° if skeletally mature
- Bracing if 25–40° during growth
- Consider operative management if Cobb angle >45° during growth or >50° if skeletally mature

JUVENILE IDIOPATHIC ARTHRITIS (JIA)

This is a type of autoimmune arthritis presenting <16 years.

Clinical features:

- Joint swelling and erythema
- Morning stiffness
- Lymphadenopathy
- Systemic upset, e.g. fever, iridocyclitis, rash

Examination:

- Swollen erythematous joints
- Limp
- Extra-articular features including rash (migratory light pink rash on trunk or extremities), lymphadenopathy, hepatosplenomegaly, cervical spine involvement

The different subtypes and their features are summarised in Table 10.1.

Investigations:

- Bloods: Full blood count (FBC), urea and electrolytes (U&Es), C-reactive protein (CRP), erythrocyte sedimentation rate (ESR),

Table 10.1 Subtypes of juvenile idiopathic arthritis and their features

Subtype	Features
Oligoarticular	Most common ≤4 joints – predominantly medium and large joints Age 1–6 years Associated with DR8 and DR5
Polyarticular	≥5 joints – predominantly small and medium joints Age 1–4 and 7–10 years Associated with DR4
Systemic (including Still disease) Worst prognosis	Rash Fevers Hepatosplenomegaly or lymphadenopathy Age 5–10 years

rheumatoid factor (seropositive in <15%), antinuclear antibody (ANA)
- X-rays of peripheral joints and/or cervical spine: may show soft tissue swelling, osteopenia, joint space narrowing, erosions

Management:

- 50% resolve, 25% ongoing symptoms, 25% severe symptoms
- Definitively rule out infection before making diagnosis
- Rheumatology referral for disease-modifying anti-rheumatic drug (DMARD) workup and ongoing management

GAIT ABNORMALITIES

Child with a limp

There are a range of causes for a limp in a child, ranging from benign to more serious ones. Note, smaller children may present with an unwillingness to weight bear, so a high index of suspicion is required. Whilst the hip is the most common source, pain is often referred to the knee and examination should be thorough and include the whole musculoskeletal system including spine and pelvis. Also consider the abdomen and inguinoscrotal region as part of your wider differential diagnosis.

Differential diagnoses should consider the age of the patient:

<3 years:
- Infection: Septic arthritis, osteomyelitis, discitis
- Toddler's fracture or stress fracture
- Developmental dysplasia of the hip (DDH) – assess for leg length discrepancy and restricted hip abduction
- Non-accidental injury, especially in non-mobile children
- Neuromuscular disease, cerebral palsy, malignancy

3–10 years:
- Transient synovitis – ask for preceding viral illness, children are normally afebrile with no restriction of ROM
- Perthes' disease – reduced ROM in hip, pain in the hip or knee, signs of synovitis, leg length discrepancy
- Infection: Septic arthritis osteomyelitis
- Traumatic injuries to bone or soft tissue
- JIA
- Leukaemia

10–19 years:
- Slipped upper femoral epiphysis (SUFE)
- Legg-Calve-Perthes (Perthes) disease
- Rheumatological: JIA, ankylosing spondylitis
- Infection: Septic arthritis, osteomyelitis, sexually transmitted
- Malignancy

Investigations:

- Observations should be taken such as heart rate (HR), blood pressure (BP), oxygen saturations, temperature and you could also consider the following depending on the clinical picture:
  - Bloods (FBC, U&E, ESR, CRP and blood culture)
  - Imaging (plain X-ray including frog-lateral of hip if SUFE, and/or hip US to look for effusion). Further imaging such as MRI/or CT may also be considered depending on working diagnosis

Kocher's criteria can help to differentiate between transient synovitis and septic arthritis in children (1):

- Non-weight bearing
- A history of fever/temperature >38.5°
- ESR > 40
- White cell count (WCC) > 12

The probability of septic arthritis is estimated as follows: 3% if one criterion, 40% if two criteria, 93% if three criteria and 99.96% if four criteria satisfied.

Non-antalgic gait

There are several different types of non-antalgic gait with potential underlying aetiologies:

1. Equinus gait or 'tiptoeing'
   - Cerebral palsy – spasticity, 'scissoring' gait due to adductor spasm, up going plantars and other upper motor neuron signs
   - Muscular dystrophy – hip girdle weakness, Gower's sign +
   - Autistic spectrum disorder – look for stereotyped or repetitive motor movements, use of objects or speech (e.g. hand flapping, echolalia) and deficits in verbal and non-verbal social communication
   - Spina bifida – associated with lower spinal pathology, abnormal neurology and muscle weakness
   - Habitual, non-pathological, toe walking is common in children and can be corrected on request
2. Spastic gait – stiff, foot dragging with foot inversion
   - Upper motor neuron lesions, e.g. diplegic or quadriplegic cerebral palsy
   - Stroke
3. Circumduction gait – excessive hip abduction as the leg swings forward
   - Leg length discrepancy
   - JIA
   - Hemiplegic cerebral palsy
4. Trendelenberg gait – pelvis fails to remain neutral in single leg stance and displays a downward tilt towards unaffected side due to weakness of hip abductors or pain
   - Perthes disease
   - SUFE
   - DDH
5. Stepping gait – associated with weak ankle dorsiflexors, hip and knee flex excessively to allow toes to clear the ground
   - Lower motor neuron (LMN) neurological disease, e.g. spina bifida, poliomyelitis
   - Peripheral neuropathies, e.g. Charcot-Marie-tooth
6. In-toeing is a normal finding in many children, and generally corrects by age 7
   - Possible causes include femoral anteversion, internal tibial torsion and metatarsus adductus. Orthopaedic referral should be considered if unilateral, painful or with a fixed metatarsus adductus (not passively correctable)

A full pregnancy, birth, developmental and general history should be sought including delay or regression of motor milestones. A family history, travel history and red flags and systemic upset should be specifically asked about.

Examination should include a gait assessment, full examination including musculoskeletal and neurological exam.

Investigations will depend on the history and examination but may include bloods (FBC, U&E, CRP, ESR, bone profile, autoantibodies, creatine kinase [CK] and blood cultures), imaging such as baseline X-rays and genetic testing via a genetic counsellor.

PARA-ATHLETES

Para-athletes are at higher risk for certain injuries depending on their classification. In general, wheelchair athletes primarily experience upper limb injury, including cervical and thoracic spine involvement, whilst ambulatory athletes tend to have lower limb injuries, including lumbar spine involvement. Overuse injuries are also common, as are alterations in bone mineral density. Gain an understanding of the athlete's classification and the demands of their sport. Any athlete with prostheses should be diligently assessed for stump or socket problems and correct prosthetic fit. Specific points to consider in limb deficient athletes:

- Prosthetic history: Skin breakdown, stump pain, prior injuries
- Inspection of stump for skin changes, reduced sensation
- Check prosthetic fit, e.g. observe gait with prosthetic on

For athletes with a spinal cord injury (SCI), it is worth familiarising yourself with the American Spinal Cord Injury Association (ASIA) classification (2) (Figures 10.5a and b). Autonomic dysreflexia, a medical emergency seen in patients with spinal cord injuries above level T6, is summarised in the Chapter 16. Finally, psychological aspects should be explored.

LEG PAIN IN A LIMB-DEFICIENT ATHLETE

"A 32-year-old, 400 metre sprinter has been referred to you with leg pain. He describes a 2-week history of shooting pain down his right leg and difficulty sleeping due to this. He reports no acute injury. He has a right below knee amputation and uses a blade prosthesis for competition. Please assess and discuss your differential diagnosis and investigations."

Differential diagnosis:

- Lumbar spine radiculopathy
- Overuse injury, e.g. hamstring origin tendinopathy

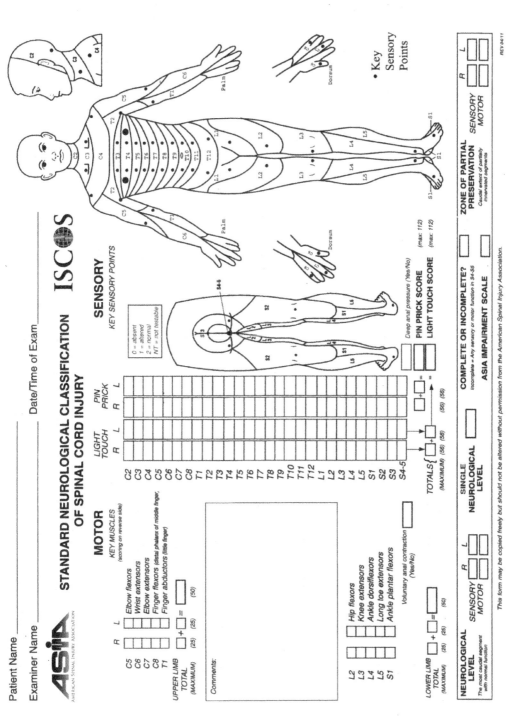

Figure 10.5 (a) American Spinal Cord Injury Association (ASIA) classification and (b) flowchart for determining the classification of individuals with SCI. (Reference Journal.) (Continued)

Appendix 2: Steps in Classification

The following order if recommended in determining the classification of individuals with SCI.

1. Determine sensory levels for right and left sides.

2. Determine motor levels for right and left sides.

   Note: in regions where there is no myotome to test, the motor level is presumed to be the same as the sensory level, if testable motor function above that level is also normal.

3. Determine the single neurological level.

   This is the lowest segment where motor and sensory function is normal on both sides, and is the most cephalad of the sensory and motor levels determined in steps 1 and 2.

4. Determine whether the injury is Complete or Incomplete (i.e. absence or presence of sacral sparing)

   If voluntary anal contraction = No AND all S4-5 sensory scores = 0 AND deep anal pressure = No, then injury is COMPLETE. Otherwise, injury is Incomplete.

5. Determine ASIA Impairment Scale (AIS) Grade:

   Is injury Complete?   If YES, AIS = A and can record ZPP (lowest dermatome or myotome on each side

   NO ⟶ with some preservation)

   Is injury motor Incomplete?   **If NO, AIS = B**

   YES ⟶ (Yes = voluntary anal contraction OR motor function more than 3 levels below the motor level on a given side, if the patient has sensory incomplete classification.)

   Are at least half of the key muscles below the single neurological level graded 3 or better?

   NO ⟶   YES ⟶

   AIS = C   AIS = D

   If sensation and motor function is normal in all segments, AIS = E

   Note: AIS E is used on follow-up testing when an individual with a documented SCI has recovered normal function. If at initial testing no deficits are found, the individual is neurologically intact; the ASIA Impairment Scale does not apply.

Figure 10.5 (*Continued*)

- Contracture
- Stump specific problems: Skin breakdown, fungal infections, neuroma, verrucous hyperplasia, heterotopic ossification, oedema causing poor prosthetic fit (especially in competitions in hot climates and after long haul flights)
- Osteomyelitis or cellulitis secondary to stump skin breakdown
- Phantom limb pain

Examination:

- Observe gait with prosthesis on and look for asymmetry of gait
- Screen lumbar spine and hip
- Perform slump or straight leg raise (SLR) if suspected lumbar spine radiculopathy
- Skin and stump examination particularly looking for skin breakdown, potential nidus of infection, spreading erythema
- Neurological exam
- Rule out cauda equina syndrome

Investigations:

- Observations: HR, BP, oxygen saturations, temperature (any signs of sepsis?)
- Bloods: Bone profile and vitamin D, FBC, U&E, CRP if suspected soft tissue or bone infection
- Consider DEXA scan to determine bone mineral density
- X-ray +/− MRI if evidence of radiculopathy or to rule our possible cauda equina syndrome (secondary to osteopenic wedge fracture of spine)
- X-ray or MRI to assess for suspected osteomyelitis of the stump

Management will depend on the diagnosis, but consider:

- Vitamin D and calcium replacement if deficient
- Tissue viability referral if skin breakdown +/− treatment for local infection, e.g. fungal
- Re-assessment for prosthetic fit and biomechanics
- Clinical psychologist involvement as part of multidisciplinary team (MDT) care

MEDICAL MUSCULOSKELETAL MASQUERADERS

ACUTE ATRAUMATIC ARTHRITIS

"This 27-year-old hockey player has recently returned from tour abroad and presents with an atraumatic painful effusion of his right knee. Please take a history and discuss your differential diagnosis and investigations."

The differential diagnosis dependent on joint involvement is summarised in Table 10.2.

There are some key questions you *must* ask in the history:

- Symptoms of inflammatory bowel disease (IBD) such as bloody diarrhoea, weight loss, mouth ulcers – enteric arthropathy
- Skin problems, e.g. psoriasis – psoriatic arthropathy
- Lower back pain (LBP) and stiffness +/− inflamed eyes (anterior uveitis), Achilles tendinopathy – ankylosing spondylitis
- History of dysuria, discharge/pelvic pain or diarrhoea – associated with sexually transmitted infections (STIs) or gastrointestinal acute infection in reactive arthritis, e.g. campylobacter. If positive, sensible to take a sexual history – reactive arthritis.
- Systemic upset and fever – septic arthritis

Examination:

- Assess for plaques of psoriasis in hairline
- Assess eyes for anterior uveitis
- Assess temperature of knee, size of effusion and ROM
- Any evidence of enthesitis, e.g. Achilles tendon

Investigations:

- Observations including HR, BP, temperature, oxygen saturations – ensure not septic
- Bloods to include:
  - FBC, U&E, LFTs, CRP, ESR and blood culture
  - HLA-B27, anti-CCP, urate

Table 10.2 Differential diagnosis of acute atraumatic arthritis

Monoarticular	Polyarticular	Lower back pain
Septic arthritis	Rheumatoid arthritis (especially if symmetric of small joints)	Axial spondyloarthropathy
Reactive arthritis	Systemic lupus erythematosus (SLE)	Psoriatic arthritis
Psoriatic arthritis	Inflammatory OA	Enteropathic arthritis
Crystal arthritis	Polyarticular gout	Reactive arthritis
Osteoarthritis (OA)	Enteropathic polyarthritis (associated with inflammatory bowel disease)	
Monoarticular rheumatoid arthritis		

- Joint aspirate: Send for cell count, differential, glucose, crystals, culture and sensitivities.
- If appropriate: Stool culture, urine culture, swabs for STIs – gonococcus, chlamydia, campylobacter
- Consider X-rays if polyarticular picture to look for marginal erosions

Reactive arthritis

The antiquated term 'Reiter's disease' referred to a clinical triad of urethritis, arthritis and conjunctivitis occurring after a gastrointestinal or genitourinary infection. Enthesopathy of the Achilles tendon and plantar fascia are common. Males are affected more commonly than females and the typical age of presentation is 20–40 years.

The knee and ankle joints are most commonly involved. Episodes last weeks to months, but some may have recurrent attacks

Common pathogens: *Shigella, Salmonella, Campylobacter, Chlamydia*

Clinical features:

- Large joint effusion
- Conjunctivitis
- Enthesopathy
- Dermatological manifestations may include keratoderma blennorrhagicum

Investigations: As above. HLA-B27 positive in 75% cases, isolate organisms from stool or urine culture. X-rays may show sacroiliac inflammation or erosive arthritis in peripheral joints.

Management: Antibiotics sensitive to organism. The vast majority are successfully treated with a course of antibiotics. Some may go on to develop a chronic inflammatory picture with intermittent and prolonged symptoms and should be referred to rheumatology for considerations of DMARDs.

SERONEGATIVE SPONDYLOARTHROPATHY

"A 23-year-old volleyball player has been referred by his GP for an insidious onset of lower back pain. He describes it worse when he wakes up, and says it takes a while 'to get going'. He has suffered from 'Achilles problems' on and off for many years. His mother has Crohn's disease."

Spectrum of inflammatory pathologies which consist of:

- Ankylosing spondylitis
- Reactive arthritis
- Psoriatic arthritis
- Enteropathic arthritis (associated with Inflammatory bowel disease)

The disease can be axial (limited to the spine and sacroiliac joints) and/or peripheral. Older texts state this is a disease of young males with HLA-B27 positivity. However, this is now outdated, and in recent years studies have reported nearly equivalent prevalence in females. It is recognised that there are sex differences in presentation of SpA between males and females. Females are more likely to be HLA-B27 negative, have non-radiographic SpA and a lower radiological progression. However, women with axial SpA show significantly lower anti-TNF efficacy and disease burden is equal between the sexes (3).

Clinical features: *Specifically ask about these in the history*

- Inflammatory back pain (or buttock pain)
  - Insidious onset
  - Age of onset <45 years
  - Duration >3 months
  - Associated with morning stiffness >30 minutes
  - Improves with exercise
- Extra-articular manifestations
  - Enthesopathies (e.g. Insertional tendinopathies – Achilles, plantar fascia, gluteal tendons)
  - Anterior uveitis (also strongly associated with HLA-B27)
  - Aortic root abnormalities
  - Dactylitis
  - Psoriasis
  - Symptoms of IBD
  - Dysuria, urethritis, cervicitis or recent acute diarrhoeal episode
- Positive family history
- Responds to NSAIDs

Classification of axial spondyloarthropathy: Assessment of SpondyloArthritis international Society (ASAS) Classification criteria for axial spondyloarthritis (4) (See box).

> Patients with ≥3 months back pain and age of onset <45 years with:
>
> Sacroiliitis on imaging and ≥1 SpA feature
>
> **OR**
>
> HLA-B27 positive and ≥2 other SpA features

SpA features: Inflammatory back pain, arthritis, enthesitis, uveitis, dactylitis, psoriasis, Crohn's/colitis, good response to NSAIDs, family history of SpA, HLA-B27, elevated CRP.

Sacroiliitis on imaging: Active inflammation on MRI suggestive of sacroiliitis, definite radiographic sacroiliitis according to modified New York criteria (5).

Note: These are classification criteria originally aimed to facilitate research in the disease and should not be used solely for diagnostic purposes. Diagnosis should be based on a combination of clinical, laboratory and imaging features by a specialist rheumatologist.

Examination:

- Examine for plaque of psoriasis and manifestations of IBD
- Loss of lumbar lordosis
- Reduced ROM lumbar flexion and lateral flexion (lateral flexion is often first to be reduced)
- Increased occiput to wall distance
- Schober's test <5 cm increase on flexion
- Reduced chest expansion and prominent abdomen
- State you would like to complete the examination by assessing the eyes for anterior uveitis, auscultate the heart for aortic incompetence, and auscultate the lungs for apical fibrosis

Investigations:

- Bloods: HLA-B27 (negative HLA-B27 does not rule out diagnosis). Note CRP and ESR are rarely significantly raised in axial disease alone
- Other (dependent on history): Rheumatoid factor, anti-CCP, fecal calprotectin, urine or stool culture (organisms involved in reactive arthritis)
- Imaging:
  a. X-rays likely to be negative if early
  b. MRI using SpA sequencing protocol such as fat-suppressed T2WI or high-resolution STIR will show active inflammation suggestive of sacroiliitis +/− corner lesions
     - MRI acute: oedema at anterior and posterior corners of vertebral body (low T1WI, high T2WI; see Chapter 18)
     - MRI chronic: Fatty replacement (High T1WI and T2WI), sclerosis (low signal T1WI and T2WI)
  c. US if any active enthesitis

Management:

1. Referral to rheumatologist
2. Exercise and physiotherapy referral
3. NSAIDs for symptomatic control initially and assess response
4. Disease modifying anti-rheumatic drugs (DMARDs), e.g. methotrexate, sulfasalazine are only effective in peripheral disease and not axial disease
5. Biologics, e.g. anti-TNF and IL-17 inhibitors if failure of 2× NSAIDs, e.g. infliximab, adalimumab
   a. Reassess after 12 weeks for a 50% reduction in Bath Ankylosing Spondylitis Disease Activity Index (BASDAI) score
   b. Side effects include reactivation of tuberculosis, hepatitis B and C: A baseline X-ray and bloods need to be performed prior to initiation of treatment. Other risks include increased risk of lymphoma and skin cancer so appropriate counselling for this should be undertaken
6. Ophthalmology referral if anterior uveitis
7. If evidence of ankylosis, then may be restrictions on contact sport as risk of fragility fractures

THE HYPERMOBILE PATIENT

"An 18-year-old swimmer presents with bilateral shoulder pain. On closer questioning she also complains of frequently having her shoulder 'pop out' of the socket, and says she has always been double-jointed. Please take and history and examine this patient."

Differential diagnosis:

- Benign joint hypermobility syndrome
- Marfan's syndrome
- EDS (hypermobility type – formally type III)
- Osteogenesis imperfecta
- Pseudoxanthoma elasticum

a. Benign joint hypermobility syndrome (BJHS)

Asymptomatic generalised joint hypermobility is common and not pathological. BJHS is a connective tissue disorder in which the individual is hypermobile and musculoskeletal symptoms are experienced in the absence of systemic rheumatological disease.

Clinical features:

- Musculoskeletal pain in multiple joints
- Hypermobility
- Fatigue
- Dysautonomia, e.g. orthostatic intolerance, headache, abdominal or pelvic pain, anxiety or depression

Examination:

- >4/9 Beighton score to examine for hypermobility
- Examine joints for swelling, correctable deformities
- Assess for skin abnormalities, e.g. hyperextensibility

Diagnosis is based on the Brighton criteria (6):

- Two major criteria
- One major and two minor criteria

- Four minor criteria or
- Two minor criteria and unequivocally affected first degree relative
  Major criteria:
  - Beighton score >4
  - Polyarthralgias: pain >3 months in 4 or more joints
  Minor criteria:
  - Beighton score <4
  - Oligoarthralgias: pain >3 months in 1–3 joints or back pain >3 months
  - Dislocation or subluxation
  - Soft tissue lesion, e.g. tenosynovitis
  - Marfanoid habitus: armspan > height (>1.03 ratio) or arachnodactyly
  - Skin abnormalities: Striae, hyperextensibility, thin skin, abnormal scarring
  - Ocular: Drooping eyelids, myopia
  - Varicosities, herniae or uterine/rectal prolapse
  - Mitral valval prolapse

Investigations: Diagnosis is clinical

Management:

- Education about condition – provide written information and signpost to helpful websites
- Taping and bracing may assist in preventing subluxations
- Physiotherapy referral for specific strengthening exercises and postural correction dependent on clinical presentation
- Analgesia, e.g. NSAIDs during flares
- Cognitive behavioural therapy may be suitable for some

b. Marfan's syndrome
Autosomal dominant connective tissue disorder due to mutations in the *FBN1* gene encoding fibrillin.
Revised Ghent nosology for diagnosis (7).

Characterised by:

- Three clinical criteria: Thoracic aortic aneurysm and/or dissection, ectopia lentis and systemic features, and
- Two genetic criteria: Presence of a first degree relative with Marfan's syndrome diagnosed according to Ghent-2 criteria and presence of a pathogenic mutation in *FBN1* gene in presence of thoracic aortic aneurysm or ectopia lentis

Diagnosis is based on the detection of

- Two of the three clinical criteria or
- One of the clinical criteria plus a family history or
- Presence of thoracic aortic aneurysm or ectopia lentis with *FBFN1* mutation

Clinical features:

- Tall and slim body habitus (Marfanoid)
- Generalised joint hypermobility
- Arachnodactyly
- Scoliosis >20°
- Myopia
- Pectus excavatum or carinatum
- Ectopia lentis

Examination:

- Increased arm span: Height or reduced upper segment/lower segment
- High arched palate, Steinberg sign and Walker-Murdoch sign+ (arachnodactyly), scoliosis
- Pes planus
- Pectus carinatum or excavatum
- Murmur secondary to mitral valve prolapse (MVP) or aortic regurgitation
- Neurological exam: Dural ectasia

Investigations:

- Electrocardiogram (ECG) and Echocardiogram
- CXR +/− cardiac and lumbosacral MRI

Management:

- Referral to geneticist for workup and genetic counselling
- Ocular examination
- Cardiology referral
- Education regarding participation in physical activity: Avoiding Valsalva, certain contact sports

c. Ehlers-Danlos syndrome (EDS) – hypermobility type
A group of inherited connective tissue disorders characterised by joint laxity, skin hyperelasticity and skin fragility. It is inherited in an autosomal dominant fashion and is due to a defect in collagen.

There are six different types of EDS (classic, hypermobile, vascular, kyphoscoliosis, arthrochalasia and dermatosparaxis) of which hypermobility type (formerly type III) is the most common.

Clinical features:

- Easy bruising, shoulder instability
- "Just **GAPE**" – Joints and other soft tissues, gut, allergy, postural symptoms, exhaustion
- Ask about family history

Examination: Focus on facial, musculoskeletal and dermatological examination

- Pigmented scars over bony prominences
- Joint hypermobility and instability
- Pes planus
- Kyphosis or scoliosis

- Soft velvety and hyperextensible skin, wide atrophic scars, pseudo-tumours (classical type)
- Other: Mitral valve prolapse, herniae, aortic aneurysm

Management:

- Referral to geneticist for genetic testing and diagnosis
- Counselling regarding pregnancy as high risk of premature rupture of membranes and postpartum haemorrhage
- Physiotherapy referral for specific strengthening exercises and proprioceptive training +/– consideration of splints, taping or braces to symptomatic joints
- Collision/contact sports should be avoided in those with vascular type EDS and certain severe forms of other types
- Surgical referral if recurrent shoulder instability

Referral to rheumatologist if any of the below features:

- Skin features, e.g. abnormal scars
- Vascular phenomena, e.g. abnormal bruises
- Facies
- Scoliosis
- Marfanoid facies + abnormal echo or lens signs
- Family history of vascular phenomena, PNX
- Ongoing MSK symptoms despite conservative management

d. Other

Pseudoxanthoma elasticum (PXE) – autosomal recessive connective tissue disorder characterised by fragile calcified vessels which rupture in skin, cardiovascular system and retina. Ask about upper gastrointestinal bleeds or haemoptysis. Angioid streaks on fundoscopy.

Osteogenesis imperfecta – often autosomal dominant characterised by reduced collaged type 1 and severely brittle bones. Several different types with varying clinical presentations. Patients have blue sclera (due to scleral thinness allowing choroid vessels to be seen), hearing impairment and easy bruising.

MALIGNANCY

Benign and malignant tumours of bone and soft tissue share a common clinical, radiological and pathological presentation. Primary malignant bone tumours include osteosarcoma, chrondrosarcoma, Ewing's sarcoma and soft-tissue sarcomas and have a preponderance for long bones of the lower limb, particularly around the knee. Benign tumours are those that does not invade surrounding tissue or spread elsewhere and include osteoid osteomas, osteochondroma or simple bone cysts. Bone metastases are common from bronchus, breast, prostate, kidney and thyroid primary sites.

Clinical features:

- Incidental finding,
- Night pain,
- Pain not responding to analgesia,
- Referred pain, e.g. pelvic tumour can refer to abdomen, back or leg,
- Progressive neurological dysfunction,
- Swelling,
- Pathological fracture.
- Painless, enlarging mass if soft-tissue sarcoma
- Screen for B symptoms including fever, weight loss, night sweats, ask about breast lumps

Examination:

- Swelling and tenderness over affected bone.
- Systemic findings rare.
- All superficial soft-tissue lesions >5 cm and all deep-seated lesions should be considered a sarcoma until proven otherwise

Investigations:

- X-rays, radionuclide scanning, CT, MRI to delineate lesion
- Benign tend to be well-demarcated while ill-defined lesions are more likely to be malignant or metastatic
- Consider staging using CT chest, abdomen, pelvis (CAP), myeloma screen, bone profile including alkaline phosphatase (ALP), PTH, CRP and ESR as infection can mimic malignancy
- Biopsy – fluoroscopic or CT guided
- Bone tumour mimics: Soft-tissue haematoma, myositis ossificans, infection, crystal arthritis
- Specific bone tumours have been described below

Osteosarcoma

This is the most common primary malignant bone tumour with a bimodal distribution peaking in adolescence and the seventh decade of life.

Clinical features:

- The majority present at the distal femur, proximal tibia or humerus
- Worsening pain, particularly night pain
- Swelling
- Skin may be warm with venous engorgement
- Pathological fracture is rare

Investigations:

- Elevated ALP and lactate dehydrogenase (LDH)
- X-rays are generally diagnostic demonstrating ill-defined, permeative bone forming lesions with cortical destruction, periosteal reaction and soft-tissue expansion. Rapidly enlarging subperiosteal lesions may elevate the periosteum so quickly that bone deposition occurs only at the margins, creating Codman's triangle. Attempts at bone formation may produce streaks of calcification termed sunray spicules (see Chapter 18)
- MRI of the whole bone will delineate medullary and extra-osseous extent of the tumour
- CT chest for lung metastases
- Biopsy of the lesion for histology

Management: Referral to sarcoma unit for MDT assessment of treatment options

Osteoid osteoma

These are small, benign tumours formed of osteoid and woven bone surrounded by a halo of reactive bone. They are common in young patients and more common in men than women.

Clinical features:

- Common in long bones
- Pain which is classically worse at night
- Pain relieved by NSAIDs
- If close to a joint: stiffness +/− effusion
- If present in the spine: muscle spasm and scoliosis

Investigations:

- X-rays demonstrate an area of dense sclerosis with a small, rounded area of osteolysis which may be obscured by surrounding sclerosis (see Chapter 18)
- CT: The central nidus of the lesion is best seen on CT scan
- Biopsy of the lesion for histology

Management: Although lesions regress over time, the preferred treatment is CT-guided radiofrequency ablation

Aneurysmal bone cyst

These are benign expansile lesions of bone composed of blood-filled cystic spaces. They can be destructive and result in significant dysfunction. They predominantly affect children and adolescents.

Clinical features:

- Commonly seen in the metaphyses of long bones, particularly the femur, tibia and humerus or posterior elements of the spine
- Pain and swelling
- If affecting the spine, they can present with nerve root impingement or neurological impairment

Investigations:

- X-rays will show a subperiosteal, poorly defined osteolytic lesion, elevating and progressively eroding the cortex
- MRI will show typical cystic features with multiple intralesional septations +/− fluid levels

Management:

- Curettage of the lesion at the time of biopsy can be effective, although recurrence is 20%
- Radiotherapy can also be effective but must be used in caution given secondary risk of malignancy or growth arrest

OSTEOMYELITIS

Acute osteomyelitis in adults can occur following an open injury, a surgical procedure or via contiguous spread, e.g. diabetic foot ulcer. Haematogenous osteomyelitis may present in the vertebrae. If a long bone is affected, it can spread within the medullary cavity and cortex and extend into surrounding soft tissues and possibly an adjacent joint.

Risk factors for bone infection:

- Malnutrition
- Diabetes mellitus
- Corticosteroids
- Immunosuppression
- Peripheral vascular disease
- Sensory peripheral neuropathy
- Trauma
- Intravenous drug use

Clinical features:

- Pain
- Fever
- Recent history of infection or procedure
- Possible local swelling and erythema

Investigations:

- Observations: Including temperature
- Bloods: FBC, U&E, LFT, CRP, ESR, blood cultures
  - Typical picture is an elevated WCC, ESR and CRP
- Imaging:
  - X-ray: May be normal during the first week, findings may include periosteal new bone formation and bone destruction (late sign) (Chapter 18)
  - CT can demonstrate bone destruction

- Radionuclide scanning is a sensitive investigation but has relatively low specificity
- MRI can be useful when the diagnosis is in doubt
- Gold standard investigation is via aspirating fluid from the metaphyseal abscess or adjacent soft tissues and sent for microscopy, culture and sensitivities (MC&S) and gram stain. The most common organism is *Staphylococcus aureus* across all ages

Management:

- Early empirical antibiotics with subsequent tailoring according to organisms identified and sensitivities. Intravenous flucloxacillin and fusidic acid are active against *S. aureus*
- Surgical drainage may be necessary

REFERENCES

1. Kocher MS, Mandiga R, Zurakowski D, Barnewolt C, Kasser JR. Validation of a clinical prediction rule for the differentiation between septic arthritis and transient synovitis of the hip in children. *J Bone Joint Surg Am.* 2004;86:1629–35.
2. Kirshblum SC, Burns SP, Biering-Sorensen F, Donovan W, Graves DE, Jha A, et al. International standards for neurological classification of spinal cord injury (revised 2011). *J Spinal Cord Med.* 2011;34(6):535–46.
3. Rusman T, van Bentum RE, van der Horst-Bruinsma IE. Sex and gender differences in axial spondyloarthritis: Myths and truths. *Rheumatology (Oxford, England).* 2020;59(Suppl4):iv38–iv46.
4. Rudwaleit M, van der Heijde D, Landewé R, Listing J, Akkoc N, Brandt J, et al. The development of Assessment of SpondyloArthritis international Society classification criteria for axial spondyloarthritis (part II): Validation and final selection. *Ann Rheumat Dis.* 2009;68:777–83.
5. van der Linden S, Valkenburg HA, Cats A. Evaluation of diagnostic criteria for ankylosing spondylitis. A proposal for modification of the New York criteria. *Arthrit Rheumat.* 1984;27(4):361–8.
6. Grahame R, Bird HA, Child A. The revised (Brighton 1998) criteria for the diagnosis of benign joint hypermobility syndrome (BJHS). *J Rheumatol.* 2000;27(7):1777–9.
7. Loeys BL, Dietz HC, Braverman AC, Callewaert BL, De Backer J, Devereux RB, et al. The revised Ghent nosology for the Marfan syndrome. *J Med Genet.* 2010;47(7):476–85.

PART B

Communication stations

INTRODUCTION

Athletes commonly present to medical care with a plethora of general medical concerns in any of the major systems. These stations have tended to have a focus on history taking, formulating a differential diagnosis and an explanation of the investigations and management with the patient and/or examiner. History taking is an art which is acquired with practice and experience. Nevertheless, this chapter will help you organise your approach to each common symptom or presentation, select a focussed battery of questions and narrow down the possible differentials. In sport and exercise medicine, you often be in an out of hospital setting. Consider if the patient in front of you requires admission to hospital acutely or whether they require ongoing secondary care investigations and management. Utilising and liaising with colleagues in other specialties and the wider MDT, e.g. dietician or psychologist is standard in a professional sports environment and should be considered in your management plan. Finally, if there is an underlying concern on the part of the patient, this should be carefully explored and addressed.

CLINICAL CASES

ATHLETE WITH A HISTORY OF COLLAPSE

"You are a medical officer working with a university triathlon club. One of the members, a 22-year-old male, semi-elite runner comes to see you before their Monday team training session and said he had a collapse over the weekend when out on a run. He was in the last few kilometres of his run when he suddenly blacked out with no preceding warning or symptoms. A friend he was running with witnessed it and said he didn't get up immediately, but he came round quickly with no confusion. They didn't see any seizure-like movement. His friend wanted to call an ambulance, but he insisted it was because he didn't have a proper breakfast and he feels fine now. He wants to know if he can race this coming weekend. Please assess."

This type of station is primarily about taking a thorough history and making a safe plan for appropriate investigations going forward, whilst safety netting with advice until these have been completed.

History:

History of presenting complaint:

*   Was loss of consciousness (LOC) complete with rapid onset and short duration (syncope)?
*   Did he recover spontaneously and completely (syncope) or was there a period of confusion thereafter (seizure)?
*   Was there a loss of postural tone? (syncope)
*   Prodrome: how did he feel before the collapse? Did he have chest pain, dizziness, shortness of breath (SOB), palpitations (possible cardiac/arrhythmia), nausea or sweating (neurally mediated syncope), was it a particularly hot day (vasovagal)?
*   What was he doing in the lead up to the event, e.g. properly fuelled (hypoglycaemia), alcohol bingeing the previous night (hypoglycaemia or seizure), has he been well in himself recently? Did the collapse happen when he was running (cardiac) or just after he stopped exercising (postural hypotension)
*   How did he feel after? Speed of recovery is important: syncope has a fast recovery whilst with seizure there is a prolonged period of confusion
*   Are there features of a seizure, e.g.
    *   Preceding aura: Somatosensory (olfactory, auditory or visual hallucinations), autonomic or 'psychic'
    *   Prolonged confusion, headache or transient limb weakness (Todd's paresis) after typically of duration >30 minutes

- Triggers: Lack of sleep, drugs or alcohol, hunger (hypoglycaemic seizure)
- Collateral history reporting seizure-like activity during episode, groaning noises, stiffness, eyes open or closed, tongue biting, incontinence, length of postictal phase
- Note, patients who have a vasovagal episode may twitch a little and those with ventricular fibrillation (VF)/ventricular tachycardia (VT) may also have some seizure-like activity, typically with paroxysmal torsades de pointes, which is short-lived and occurs after the LOC
- Any recent long-distance travel or immobilisation and/or calf swelling? (DVT/PE)
- A collateral history is essential and state you would seek this from his friend. Did anyone manage to video the episode?

Past medical history:

- Any previous episodes and their precipitants?
- Any genetic conditions, e.g. Marfan's syndrome (aortic dissection)
- Diabetes mellitus on insulin
- History of seizures, febrile convulsions or previous head injuries

Family history:

- Sudden cardiac death (SCD) (also ask about unexplained deaths, drowning, syncope in family)
- Coronary heart disease (CHD) (1st-degree relative male <55 years, female <65 years)
- Other: Cardiomyopathy, hypertension, Marfan's syndrome, diabetes mellitus

Drug history:

- Prescribed medications
- Over the counter (OTC) medications
- Drugs which prolong the QT interval, e.g. antimicrobials (ciprofloxacin, erythromycin, ketoconazole), antidepressants (fluoxetine, sertraline, amitriptyline), antiarrhythmics (amiodarone, sotalol), antipsychotics (haloperidol, quetiapine), other (sumatriptan)
- Recreational drugs, alcohol or performance-enhancing drugs

Examination (may be entirely normal):

- Basic observations including lying and standing blood pressure (BP), heart rate (HR), oxygen saturations, respiratory rate (RR) and blood sugar (BM)
- Particular focus on cardiovascular examination:
  - Slow rising pulse (aortic stenosis), jerky (hypertrophic cardiomyopathy [HCM])
  - Apex beat
  - Auscultation for murmurs
  - Pulses
- Any clinical features of Marfan's syndrome

Differential diagnosis:

- Cardiac syncope – bradycardia, tachyarrhythmia, structural cardiac disease, e.g. HCM, aortic stenosis, pulmonary embolism, aortic dissection
- Postural hypotension – primary or secondary autonomic failure, dehydration
- Reflex – vasovagal, situational, e.g. cough, micturition, carotid sinus syncope (collapse after turning head)
- Seizure
- Hypoglycaemia

Management: discussion with the patient

- Explain the possible diagnosis to the patient. In the case above, there was a syncopal episode during exercise with no preceding prodrome, so cardiac abnormalities must be ruled out in the first instance.
- Advise the patient not to drive (as per the Driver and Vehicle Licensing Agency [DVLA] https://www.gov.uk/government/publications/assessing-fitness-to-drive-a-guide-for-medical-professionals), swim or cycle until further investigations are completed to prevent them and others from serious harm should they have a further episode
- They must refrain from physical activity until their investigations are completed and reviewed by a physician, so they cannot compete in this weekend's race

Further investigations:

- Depending on the setting you are in, there may be limited resources to perform further investigations. The patient should be referred to secondary care for semi-urgent further investigations, e.g. ambulatory care unit with referral letter
- Suggested investigations would depend on the history. Initial investigations would include bloods (full blood count [FBC], urea and electrolytes [U&E], liver function tests [LFTs[, bone profile, glucose), a 12-lead electrocardiogram (ECG), echocardiography, 7-day ECG monitoring +/– exercise stress test, tilt-table testing. Cardiology investigations, e.g. ECG and echocardiogram should be interpreted by a cardiologist.
- If history is more suggestive of a seizure, then an inpatient computed tomography (CT) scan of the head is recommended with referral to first-fit clinic with outpatient magnetic

resonance imaging (MRI) scan of the head and an electroencephalogram (EEG).

RELATIVE ENERGY DEFICIENCY IN SPORT (RED-S)

"You have been asked to review a 21-year-old university cyclist who has come to see you as she is concerned with the irregularity of her periods. She had a delayed menarche at 16 and has approximately 5 periods per year which are very light. Her current BMI is 17.9. She would like to discuss starting the combined oral contraceptive (cOCP) to regulate her periods. Please take a history and discuss your investigations and management plan with her."

Relative energy deficiency in sport (RED-S) is a syndrome characterised by impaired physiological function including but not limited to the menstrual function, bone health, immunity, protein synthesis, cardiovascular health and metabolic rate secondary to relative energy deficiency (1). It can present in both males and females.

History:
Menstrual history (if female) – age of menarche, regularity of periods, duration of bleed, heaviness of periods, any previous contraception. Any periods of amenorrhoea previously?

- Amenorrhoea (no cycle for 6 months) – is it primary or secondary?
- Oligomenorrhoea (<9 cycles per year or cycle >35 days)
- Any concerning features, e.g. intermenstrual bleeding or postcoital bleeding?

Training history – including type, frequency and duration, current level of sport and ambition. Any periods of underperformance?

Nutritional history:

- Ideally, ask to see a meal plan
- Any fasted sessions, e.g. before breakfast
- Any dietary restrictions, e.g. vegan
  Eating disorder screening – e.g. SCOFF questionnaire [2]
  S – Do you make yourself SICK ...?
  C – Do you worry you have lost CONTROL?
  O – Have you recently lost more than ONE stone in 3 months?
  F – Do you believe yourself to be FAT?
  F – Would you say that FOOD dominates your life?
- Psychopathology of eating disorders (ED) including pursuit of thinness, fear of weight gain, food restriction, use of laxatives or slimming pills, bingeing or purging behaviour and any weight loss >10% in 1 month

Injury history – including stress fractures or recurrent infections/illnesses?

Ask about other features that may suggest an alternative diagnosis:

- Polycystic ovarian syndrome (PCOS) – hirsutism, weight gain, subfertility, acne
- Primary ovarian failure – strong family history, vasomotor symptoms including night sweats, previous chemotherapy

Family history: any history of primary ovarian failure

Social history

Drugs and allergies – including OTC medication or slimming aids

Differential diagnosis:

- RED-S
- Eating disorder (or disordered eating)
- PCOS
- Primary ovarian failure
- Pregnancy or breastfeeding
- Underlying medical condition, e.g. endocrine cause (17 alpha-hydroxylase deficiency)

Examination:
Are there any features of an eating disorder including parotid enlargement, lanugo hair, dry skin, cold peripheries? Any features of PCOS including hirsutism or acne?

Investigations to consider for secondary amenorrhoea

Observations: HR, BP, height and weight, body fat %

ECG – bradycardia, small QRS in anorexia nervosa

Bloods:

FBC (anaemia), U&E, LFTs, TFTs, magnesium (Mg^{2+})

Vitamin D and bone profile, iron studies and haematinics

Glucose, HBA1c, lipids (can be raised in anorexia nervosa)

Gonadotropin-releasing hormone (GnRH), follicle-stimulating hormone (FSH), luteinising hormone (LH), oestradiol, prolactin, testosterone, dehydroepiandrosterone sulphate (DHEAs), beta-HCG (see box for difference in hormonal profile in RED-S vs. PCOS)

RED-S	PCOS
↓ LH and FSH	↑ LH
↓ Oestradiol	Normal or ↓ FSH
	↑ Testosterone

Imaging:

> Dual-energy X-ray absorptiometry (DEXA) scan
> (Z score <−1.0 SD is abnormal in athletes)
> Ultrasound (US) Ovaries – PCOS

"On questioning, the patient admits that her training volume has recently increased without a corresponding increase in her food intake. She says she has 'always been thin' but that she does occasionally skip meals as she believes being slimmer will help her on hill climbs."

Management for RED-S:

1. Education:
   - It may be inadvertent undernutrition or part of an overt ED – fundamental issue is **insufficient energy availability**
   - Explain risks if untreated: osteoporosis, infertility, recurrent stress fractures, cardiac abnormalities and negative impact on performance
   - cOCP will *not* protect against bone loss – weight gain/increase in energy availability is mainstay
2. Restore energy availability
   - Dietician referral – review diet and pre-empt loading with increased nutrition
   - Training load review – may require temporary reduction of load as well as increased kcal
3. Optimise bone health
   - Vitamin D +/− calcium +/− iron supplementation if deficient or insufficient. The National Institute for Health and Care Excellence (NICE) guidance in the UK:
     - <25 nmol/L deficient – daily 4000 IU vitamin D$_3$, then 800 IU maintenance

   - 25–50 nmol/L insufficient – daily 4000 IU
   - >50 normal – maintenance in winter. Note in some elite settings 75–100 nmol/L is preferred for athletes.
   - Safe sun exposure advice, dietary advice, e.g. oily fish, eggs, meat
   - Regular resistance exercise
4. Perform RED-S triage and risk assessment according to RED-S clinical assessment tool (1, 3) (Table 11.1)

May need to instigate personalised contract with athlete involving the multidisciplinary team (MDT) (coach, psychiatrist, dietician, sports physician) with individualised requirements such as:

a. Diet plan and expected weight gain
b. Training plan
c. Therapy plan – cognitive behavioural therapy (CBT) or psychiatric involvement if disordered eating or ED

Return to training and competition is dependent on engagement and achievement of above.

Note: At the time of writing, transdermal oestradiol (given with cyclic progesterone) has had some success in increasing BMD in patients with anorexia nervosa and normal weight oligomenorrheic athletes (4). Bisphosphonates and other therapies are not recommended in premenopausal women.

UNWELL ATHLETE

"You are a doctor at a national watersports championship. An 18-year-old canoeist comes to see you 2 hours prior to their race feeling unwell with abdominal pain. They have recently returned from a holiday in Spain. On further questioning the athlete says they

Table 11.1 RED-S risk assessment and recommended management according to risk

High risk	Moderate risk	Low risk
Eating disorder, e.g. anorexia nervosa or bulimia nervosa Severe ECG abnormalities Extreme weight loss techniques with dehydration and/or haemodynamically instability Other serious medical conditions linked to RED-S	Prolonged low body fat 5–10% weight loss in 1 month Amenorrhoea or abnormal menstrual cycle Abnormal hormonal profile in men History of 1+ stress fracture associated with low energy availability Reduced BMD Behaviour affecting other team members	Normal hormonal and metabolic function Normal BMD Healthy musculoskeletal system Appropriate energy availability
No competition or training Written contract May require psychiatry referral	Training allowed under contract Competition once medical clearance	Full training and competition

BMD, bone mineral density; ECG, electrocardiogram; RED-S, relative energy deficiency in sport.

Source: Adapted from the RED-S clinical assessment tool in (1).

have lost weight and are hungry all the time. Please take a history and state what examination and investigations you would like to do."

History:

- Take a chronological history of events
- Abdominal pain — central or right iliac fossa (appendicitis or pancreatitis), right upper quadrant (cholecystitis), suprapubic (urinary tract infection, gynaecological)
- Any episodes of diarrhoea or vomiting?
- Any dysuria or polyuria: Onset, volume of urine passed, frequency, volume and colour of urine
- Appetite, weight loss
- Symptoms suggestive of an infection e.g. upper respiratory tract infection (URTI), urinary tract infection (UTI), gastrointestinal upset, e.g. food poisoning from recent travel
- Any other features which could explain symptoms, e.g. malignancy, viral infection, e.g. glandular fever (Epstein-Barr virus [EBV]), possible pregnancy

Past medical history and family history, especially autoimmune disorders

Medication history and allergies

Examination:

- General observation – hydration status e.g. skin turgor
- Cardiovascular and respiratory examination
- Abdominal examination – exclude acute abdomen
- Screen for infection – ear, nose and throat (ENT) exam, chest auscultation, palpate bladder
- State would like to do basic observations including HR, BP, temperature, oxygen saturation, RR

Investigations:

- Urine dip for nitrites, leucocytes, glucose, ketones and β-hCG
- Bloods if resources – FBC, U&E, LFTs, C-reactive protein (CRP), glucose, ketones

Differential diagnosis:

- Intra-abdominal sepsis e.g. appendicitis, cholecystitis
- Urinary tract infection
- New presentation of diabetes mellitus
- Infective gastroenteritis

"Examiner states nil on general examination apart from volume depletion.

BP is 105/65, HR is 80 bpm, temperature 37.5°, oxygen saturations 98% on air, RR is 25.

Urine dip shows glucose +++ and ketones ++."

Management and discussion

- Explain to patient that they likely have underlying type 1 diabetes causing a lack of insulin. This has caused a dangerously high blood glucose which will require admission to hospital for treatment
- Treatment acutely will include intravenous (IV) fluids, insulin and potassium replacement as well as a septic screen in hospital
- Explain that after sugars have stabilised they will require lifelong insulin treatment under a specialist
- Provide reassurance that once stabilised it is possible to live a normal life and compete with type 1 diabetes
- Be clear with patient that they are unable to compete this afternoon as their blood sugars are dangerously high
- Assist in organising their transfer to hospital with someone to accompany them, and provide proper handover
- Check the patient's understanding and ask if they would like you to inform anyone else, e.g. parents, coach
- Offer follow-up and provide contact information and document everything

RESPIRATORY – ATHLETE WITH SHORTNESS OF BREATH

"A 17-year-old elite swimmer has presented to your clinic complaining of a 4-month history of difficulty breathing, producing 'a high wheezing noise' in her throat during training sessions when exercising at high intensity. She has recently joined the national team and is struggling with the extra training sessions. She denies a fever or productive sputum and is otherwise well outside of training. Her recent spirometry results and readings are below (Figure 11.1 and Table 11.2). Please could you take a history and explain your investigations and possible management?"

Respiratory conditions in athletes are extremely common, and you should feel comfortable taking a

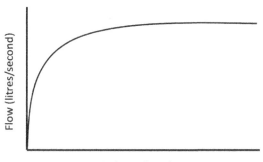

Figure 11.1 Spirometry results for patient.

Table 11.2 Spirometry results including FVC, FEV$_1$ and peak flow for patient

Parameter	Trial 1	Trial 2	Trial 3
FVC (litres)	3.99	4.01	3.98
FEV$_1$ (litres)	3.49	3.52	3.53
PEFR (litres/min)	470	475	477

FVC, forced vital capacity; FEV$_1$, forced expiratory volume; PEFR, peak flow.

history and coming up with a sensible differential diagnosis and investigation and management plan. You may also be presented with lung function or spirometry results from a patient so you should have an understanding and working knowledge of how these investigations are performed and be able to interpret a simple flow-volume loop or data.

- FEV$_1$ is the forced expiratory volume (L) in 1 second after full inspiration
- FVC (forced vital capacity) is the total volume of air which can be exhaled when blowing out as fast as possible
- PEFR (peak expiratory flow rate) is the maximal flow rate of air
- FEV$_1$/FVC ratio is the ratio of the forced expiratory volume in the first one second to the forced vital capacity of the lungs. An obstructive pattern, e.g. classically asthma, will have values <80% of predicted

Main differentials

- Exercise-induced bronchoconstriction (EIB) or asthma
- Exercise-induced laryngeal obstruction (EILO)
- Rhinosinusitis
- Gastroesophageal reflux disease (GORD)
- URTI/lower respiratory tract infection (LRTI)
- Do not miss: Cardiac pathology, pneumothorax, pulmonary embolus (PE), anaemia

Exercise-induced bronchoconstriction is characterised by inspiratory and expiratory wheeze in the chest, which is worse 30 minutes after exercise which can be associated with a post-exercise cough. It does not resolve quickly on cessation of exercise, but it responds to β$_2$ agonists.

Exercise-induced laryngeal obstruction is characterised by inspiratory stridor with associated throat tightness which peaks approximately 5 minutes into exercise and resolves quickly. It does not respond to β$_2$ agonists [5].

Chronic rhinosinusitis is characterised by nasal congestion or discharge, facial pressure and parosmia.

History:

- Symptoms to specifically ask about:
  - Wheeze
  - Stridor
  - Cough
  - Chest pain/discomfort
  - Early fatigue
    - SOB
    - Throat constriction
    - Sputum
    - Acid reflux
    - Nasal congestion
- Timing of symptoms – does it come on after exercise (EIB) or when exercising at peak intensity (EILO)?
- Resolution – do symptoms persistent after stopping exercise (EIB) or resolve rapidly after cessation of exercise (EILO)?
- Is the sound high pitched and coming from the throat on inspiration (stridor – EILO) or wheezy and on inspiration and expiration (EIB)?
- What makes the symptoms worse? EIB – cold dry air, chlorine, pollen
- Any treatments used to date? EIB will often respond to β$_2$ agonists but EILO won't

PMH: Any history of atopy including hay fever (supports EIB or asthma)

Social history – smoking history, pets, occupation

Drug history and allergies

Training history

Ideal, concerns and expectations

Examination:

- Pay particular attention to cardiac and respiratory systems
- Take basic observations including HR, BP, RR, temperature and oxygen saturations

Investigations: Consider doing the following depending on the history

1. Bloods: FBC (white cell count [WCC], haemoglobin [Hb] and eosinophils), U&E, LFT, CRP (if concerned LRTI)
2. Sputum culture (microscopy, culture and sensitivities [MC&S] and eosinophils)
3. ECG +/– echocardiography
4. Chest X-ray (CXR): Rule out pneumothorax or LRTI
5. Spirometry (including airway reversibility) +/– bronchoprovocation testing to assess for diagnosis of EIB/asthma (6) (Figures 11.2 and 11.3)
   - An obstructive pattern will have an FEV$_1$ < 80% predicted value and FEV$_1$/FEV of <0.8

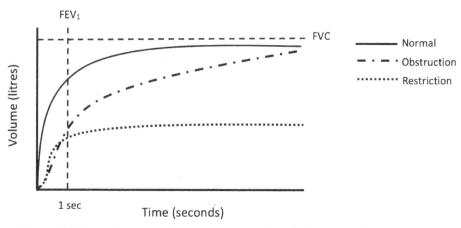

Figure 11.2 Figure demonstrating spirometry results including FVC and FEV$_1$ of normal, obstructive and restrictive patterns.

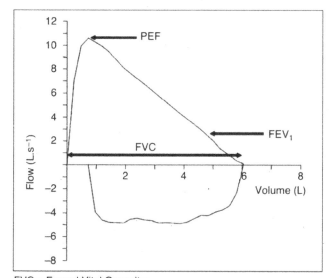

FVC = Forced Vital Capacity;
FEV$_1$ = Forced Expiratory Volume in One Second;
PEF = Peak Expiratory Flow

(a)

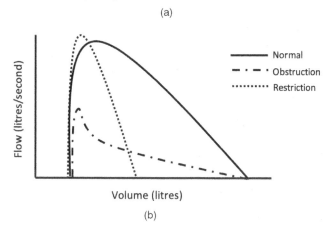

(b)

Figure 11.3 (a) Forced flow-volume loop in a normal healthy participant. (Reproduced with kind permission from the *Complete Guide to Respiratory Care in Athletes*, Routledge, 2020.) (b) Flow-volume loop representing a normal, obstructive and restrictive pattern.

- Indirect tests first line generally for EIB
  - E.g. Eucapnic voluntary hyperpnoea (EVH) – diagnosis of EIB is >10% fall in FEV_1 at two time points from baseline or
  - Osmotic challenge tests such as inhaled Mannitol – positive is 15% drop in FEV_1
- Direct tests such as methacholine useful to distinguish whether asthma or EIB
- Fractional exhaled nitric oxide (FeNO) indirect marker of airway inflammation – raised FeNO > 50 ppb has a value in detecting EIB and monitoring response to inhaled corticosteroids (ICS)
6. Continuous laryngoscopy during exercise test (invasive test)– gold standard for EILO

Management: Exercise-induced laryngeal obstruction

1. Education of condition
2. Treat any concomitant problems, e.g. hay fever
3. Refer for breathing control and diaphragmatic exercises
4. Specialist referral if refractory symptoms to respiratory specialist or ENT
5. Psychology input if required

Management: Exercise-induced bronchoconstriction (6)

1. Education
   a. Concordance to treatment essential to improve symptoms
   b. Avoiding particular triggers
   c. Reassure regarding doping guidelines (inhaled corticosteroids are permitted)
2. Pharmacotherapy including explaining correct inhaler technique
   1st line: Short-acting β_2 agonist (SABA), e.g. salbutamol 10 minutes pre-exercise
   2nd line: Regular Inhaled corticosteroid (ICS) + long-acting β_2 agonist (LABA)
   Other: Mast cell stabilisers or leukotriene inhibitor
3. Treat comorbidities
   a. Hay fever – Treat with non-sedating antihistamine or intranasal corticosteroid. Avoid oral decongestants (WADA restricted)
   b. Acid reflux
4. Other adjunctive therapies: Advise on adequate warm up, low salt diet, healthy diet rich in fruit and vegetables and omega-3, e.g. oily fish
5. Arrange follow up to check adherence to treatment and troubleshoot lack of response, e.g. poor technique. May require a repeat EVH test after 3/12 treatment

GASTROINTESTINAL – ATHLETE WITH DIARRHOEA

"A volleyball player has come to see you in clinic as they have had a 7-day history of bloody diarrhoea, abdominal cramps and fever. They can keep fluids down but they vomit if they try to eat solids at the moment. They have had some limited episodes of diarrhoea in the past but never this severe. They are in the middle of a training camp for a major competition. Please assess."

Differential diagnosis:

- Infective gastroenteritis, e.g. norovirus, campylobacter
- Inflammatory bowel disease (IBD) – Crohn's or ulcerative colitis
- Malabsorption, e.g. coeliac disease, pancreatic insufficiency
- Other: malignancy, antibiotic-associated diarrhoea, laxative abuse, thyrotoxicosis, diabetic ketoacidosis (DKA), appendicitis

History:

- Key symptoms to specifically ask about:
  - Diarrhoea
  - Vomiting
  - Fever
  - Abdominal pain
  - Weight loss
  - Mouth ulcers
  - Steatorrhoea
  - Obvious preceding food source for infection
- Frequency and timing of symptoms – how many loose motions per day
- Blood in the diarrhoea – mixed in, frank blood or melaena?
- Extraintestinal manifestations of IBD – mouth ulcers, cutaneous, e.g. erythema nodosum, arthropathy, uveitis
- Significant weight loss, tenesmus, alternating diarrhoea and constipation – malignancy
- Coeliac – diarrhoea, steatorrhoea, certain provoking foods, dermatitis herpetiformis
- Recent travel or recently eaten uncooked foods and latency of illness – infective gastroenteritis
- Other gastrointestinal symptoms: Acid reflux, dysphagia, bloating, fullness, anorexia, haematemesis, screen for systemic symptoms

PMH: IBD

Fhx: IBD, autoimmune disorders

Drug history and allergies

Social history

Examination:

Abdominal examination with particular attention paid to assess for volume depletion secondary to dehydration and extraintestinal manifestations of IBD. Assess for an acute abdomen.

Investigations: Depending on the setting

- Observations: HR, BP, temperature, oxygen saturations
- Bloods: FBC, U&E, LFTs, bone profile, CRP, haematinics and iron
- Anti-TTG
- Blood culture
- Stool culture – for organisms MC&S, fecal calprotectin, fecal elastase
- May need referral for further investigations, e.g. colonoscopy if above tests normal and chronic symptoms

Management of infective gastroenteritis in athletic setting:

1. Advise athlete to restrict training and competition until systemically well – no fever or myalgia
2. Treatment is largely supportive: advice on oral rehydration including electrolyte replacement
3. Will require to isolate during illness and for 48 hours after symptoms resolve
   - May have to liaise with coach to ensure no other athletes also have infective symptoms
4. Dietary review prior to restarting training – may be under-fuelling due to recent illness. Advise against dairy initially as may cause transient post-infective lactose intolerance
5. If athlete dehydrated, requiring IV fluids and secondary care referral will need to fill out a therapeutic use exemption (TUE)
6. Liaise with coach regarding inability to train and likely downtime
7. If notifiable organism isolated, report to national public health body, e.g. campylobacter or salmonella and inform catering team at camp
8. Education of athlete and team regarding hygiene practices including during travel

ATHLETE FATIGUE

"A 23-year-old university rower, John Smith, has been referred by his coach as he has been struggling a lot with increased fatigue after training sessions over the past 2 months. His competition times have been worsening and he has been suffering from recurrent URTIs during the season. He is studying medicine and is about to sit his fourth year exams. He has been waking up before training to do extra revision and often skips breakfast because of this. Please take a history and explain your investigations and management plan."

Unexplained underperformance syndrome (UPS) is a persistent unexplained performance deficit (recognised and agreed by coach and athlete) despite two weeks of relative rest.

Major disease should be ruled out prior to making a diagnosis of UPS. The differential diagnosis is summarised in Table 11.3.

History:

History of presenting complaint:

- Duration and pattern fatigue: Onset, duration, triggers, recent travel
- Recent illnesses and duration
- Underperformance: Quantify degree and duration, physiological measures, e.g. training HR
- Sleep: Duration and quality, insomnia, daytime naps
- Training and competition: Volume, intensity, number of competitions, recovery time

Table 11.3 Differential diagnosis for athlete fatigue according to athlete factors, medical factors and diagnoses not to miss

Athlete factors	Medical causes	Do not overlook
• Poor sleep • Undernutrition • Medications or recreational drugs • Increased training with inadequate recovery • Social factors, e.g. stress from university or relationships • Nutritional deficiency: Vitamin D, calcium, iron • Injury, e.g. MSK, concussion • Allergies	• Respiratory: Asthma, sinusitis • Gastrointestinal: Coeliac • Cardiovascular: Inherited • Endocrine: DM, hypothyroid • Rheumatological: SpA, RhA • Viral: EBV • Neurological: MS • Psychiatric comorbidity: Depression, anxiety, ED	• Pregnancy • Malignancy • Infectious disease: Malaria, HIV

DM, diabetes mellitus; ED, eating disorder; EBV, Epstein-Barr virus; HIB, human immunodeficiency virus; MS, multiple sclerosis; MSK, musculoskeletal; SpA, spondyloarthropathy.

- Nutritional history: Typical daily food and fluid intake, timing, dietary exclusions, recent changes
- Menstrual history
- Psychological screen: Low mood or anxiety, disordered eating

Past medical history: Injuries, illness, surgery

Family history: Sudden death, atopy

Social history: Current stressors including work, university, examinations, relationships, financial, support structure

Drug history: Beta blockers, antihistamines, sedatives, alcohol use, smoking, recreational drugs

Explore ideas, concerns and expectations

Systems review:

- Respiratory: Cough, wheeze, SOB
- Cardiovascular: chest pain, palpitations, syncope
- Gastrointestinal – abdominal pain, change in bowel habit, jaundice, nausea or vomiting
- Endocrine – polyuria or polydipsia, hyperthyroid symptoms (weight loss, heat intolerance, sweating, diarrhoea, oligomenorrhoea), hypothyroid (fatigue, cold intolerance, weight gain, constipation, menorrhagia)
- Rheumatological: Morning stiffness, swollen joints, skin rashes
- B symptoms: Weight loss, fever, night sweats, lymphadenopathy

Examination:

Explain what you would like to do:

Particular focus on the cardiovascular, respiratory and gastrointestinal systems

Check for lymphadenopathy

Assess for features suggesting thyroid disease

- Hyperthyroidism: Tremor, atrial fibrillation (AF), palmar erythema, lid lag, goitre, Grave's eye disease
- Hypothyroidism: Bradycardia, dry skin and hair, non-pitting oedema, slow relaxing reflexes

Investigations:

- Bedside tests: Height and weight, observations (HR, BP, temperature, O_2 saturations)
- Urine dip for BM, blood, protein, leucocytes
- ECG
- Bloods: FBC, U&E, LFTs, bone profile and vitamin D, CRP, TFTs, glucose
  - Iron studies and haematinics (B12 and folate)

Further investigations dependent on history:

- Humoral immune deficiency, e.g. IgG3

- Coeliac serology (if symptoms)
- Rheumatoid factor, anti CCP, HLA-B27
- Viral screen including EBV, cytomegalovirus (CMV), hepatitis, human immunodeficiwncy virus (HIV), antistreptolysin O (ASOT)
- FSH, LH, oestradiol, testosterone, prolactin
- Spirometry and CXR
- Echocardiogram

Management of UPS (as per the case above):

1. Education – explain likely diagnosis but need to rule out medical causes with investigations above
2. Treat any concomitant problems, e.g. hay fever
3. Start training log to monitor training and energy levels to ensure proper periodisation

Address likely underlying factors:

4. Nutrition – avoid fasted sessions, dietician review to design a programme with sufficient carbohydrate, energy and fluid. Avoid alcohol and excess caffeine
5. Poor sleep – explain basic sleep hygiene measures aiming for >8 hours per night, possibly re-planning revision timetable to ensure adequate sleep, avoid sedatives
6. Training
   a. May need 6- to 12-week period of relative rest
   b. Liaise with coach to adapt training programme: Graded exercise programme, avoid total exhaustive efforts, ensure peak training camps do not coincide with lead up to exams
7. Psychology referral if underlying mood disturbance
8. Advice on reducing stress: Mindfulness, spend time with friends, book holiday for after exams

---

Key points

- Rule out underlying medical cause
- Tailor investigations according to history
- Management requires MDT input addressing, training, diet, mood and life stressors with regular review

---

PSYCHIATRY

ALCOHOL DEPENDENCE

"You are the club doctor in a professional football team. A 35-year-old player comes to see you confidentially to discuss his poor sleep and asks if you could prescribe him a sleeping pill. He describes being unable

to get to sleep, especially after evening matches and some early morning wakening. He describes needing to drink at least a quarter to half a bottle of whisky most nights to get to sleep now, and wakes up most mornings sweaty. He feels anxious about his imminent upcoming retirement. Please take a history and explain your management for this player."

History:

History of presenting complaint:

- Sleep – explore the sleep disturbance including difficulty initiating sleep, early morning wakening, daytime somnolence, use of sleeping pills
- Alcohol history:
  - Onset and duration of increased alcohol intake
  - Assess current drinking pattern – frequency, time of day
  - Quantify alcohol intake – how much and what alcohol in an average day or week
  - Drinking behaviours – does he drink alone or with friends?
  - Signs of dependence – narrowing of drinking repertoire, withdrawal symptoms including previous seizures, requiring an eye-opener, increased tolerance.
  - Brief screening, e.g. CAGE (see box)

CAGE screening questions for alcohol misuse

C Have you ever felt that you should **C**ut down on your drinking?

A Have people **A**nnoyed you by criticising your drinking?

G Have you ever felt bad or **G**uilty about your drinking?

E Do you need a drink first thing in the morning to steady your nerves? (an **E**ye-opener)

- Psychological assessment
  - Low mood: *During the past month have you felt low, depressed or hopeless?*
  - Anhedonia: *Have you recently had little interest or pleasure in doing things?*
  - Biological symptoms: Anorexia, weight loss, difficulty concentrating, fatigue, insomnia, loss of libido
  - Thoughts of self-harm or suicide: *Have you ever thought of hurting yourself or ending your life?*
    - Ideally, a formal risk assessment should be performed including any formal plans and methods, previous

attempts, access to methods, any protective factors
- Other: Hallucinations, delusions
- Can use a validated athlete screening tool, e.g. International Olympic Committee Sport Mental Health Assessment Tool (SMHAT) (7)

Past medical history: Including previous psychiatric diagnoses, recurrent concussion

Family history: Psychiatric disorders or alcoholism

Social history: Relationships, family, financial problems, social support

Drug history: Medications, OTC or recreational

Examination: Patient should be assessed for signs of alcohol withdrawal including tremor, sweating, vomiting, confusion and consider basic observations including BP, HR, RR, oxygen saturations.

Assess gastrointestinal system for manifestations of chronic liver disease, e.g. spider naevi, ascites, jaundice, palmar erythema

Investigations: May not be required in this setting but could consider FBC, U&E, LFTs and liver screen including liver ultrasound to assess for fatty liver, fibrosis or cirrhosis.

Clinical formulation: The above patient is presenting with insomnia and features of alcohol dependence +/− concurrent mood disorder.

Management:

1. Alcohol
   a. Referral to community alcohol team to arrange formal review and management
   b. Provide information about local peer-support groups, e.g. Alcoholics Anonymous (AA)
   c. May require detox with benzodiazepine reducing regime and vitamin B replacement.
   d. Advise against the abrupt cessation of alcohol i.e. not to stop "cold turkey".
2. Mood – if a concurrent mood disorder is present:
   a. Referral to a psychologist for CBT to address low mood and anxiety
   b. Liaise with General Practitioner (GP) regarding consideration of a selective serotonin reuptake inhibitor (SSRI)
   c. May benefit from formal psychiatric referral and assessment for continuity of care
   d. Advice on accessing professional mental health resources, e.g. Professional

Football Association: Sporting Chance Clinic – current and retired athletes can self-refer for counselling and psychology input, psychiatry, funded by the Professional Football Association (PFA), players need to be a member

3. Sleep
   a. Provide sleep hygiene booklet and reinforce good practice, e.g. avoidance of visual stimulation, e.g. no television/ smart phone 2 hours prior to sleep, have a regular sleep routine, avoid excess caffeine during the day
   b. Education regarding judicial use of sleeping pills, dependence and effect on performance. Sleep disturbance, in this case likely to resolve if alcohol and mood are addressed

4. Social: Referral to local counselling service for support and arrange assessment for After Career Consultation to address concerns about upcoming retirement (8)

5. If player wants time off during treatment, explain that you can advise the coach that he cannot be selected due to medical reasons but that you don't need to divulge the reason why if he does not want you to break confidentiality

---

Key points

- Quantify alcohol use and signs of withdrawal and dependence
- Cover psychological and biological symptoms of mood disorder and always risk assess including suicidal ideation
- Support the patient with referrals to specialist resources, e.g. alcohol support and professionals, e.g. CBT or psychiatrist if necessary

---

LOW MOOD AND DELIBERATE SELF-HARM

"You are the team doctor for a gymnastics team currently abroad at a major tournament. The coach has sent a gymnast to speak to you with an unexplained headache and says he can't compete. You notice that the patient seems withdrawn and has recently lost some weight. On further questioning he admits that after the recent breakdown of his relationship with his girlfriend he has been self-harming and "just wants it all to end."

In these types of stations, attempt to establish a rapport with the patient early on and use empathic questioning, appropriate body language and periods of silence to allow them to open up. Start with open questions followed by closed questions to establish their intentions and overall risk.

History:

- Start with an open question, e.g. *Tell me how you are feeling at the moment* – allow the patient to volunteer the information
- Self-harm
  - How did you harm yourself? What did you use? How do you feel about it now? What made you harm yourself?
  - If patient admits to taking an overdose, ascertain the exact substance, quantity, route of administration, time of ingestion (and whether it was staggered) and current symptoms
  - Actions after the act – did they seek help or tell anyone
  - Expected outcome – did you think you would die?
- High-risk features
  - Planned act with precautions to prevent detection, e.g. making sure they were alone
  - Final acts, e.g. writing a note, organising finances
  - Not seeking help after act was carried out
  - Previous attempts
  - Communicating suicidal intentions
  - History of previous episodes of significant mood changes
- Current mental state
  - Low mood: *During the past month have you felt low, depressed or hopeless?*
  - Anhedonia: *Have you recently had little interest or pleasure in doing things?*
  - Biological symptoms: Anorexia, weight loss, difficulty concentrating, fatigue, insomnia, loss of libido, diurnal variation in mood
  - Any features of mania: Grandiose thoughts, insomnia, episode of feeling elated or full of energy, easily agitated, pressure of speech, history of gambling or risky behaviour
  - Other: Hallucinations, delusions
  - Can use a validated athlete screening tool, e.g. International Olympic Committee Sport Mental Health Assessment Tool (SMHAT) (7)
- Establish suicide risk
  - Should be quantified as low, medium or high. You can use validated resources to screen, e.g. the Ask Suicide-Screening Questions (ASQ) Toolkit (https://www. nimh.nih.gov/research/research-conducted-at-nimh/asq-toolkit-materials/index.shtml)

- Do they regret their actions: *'Do you still feel you want to harm yourself or end your life?'*
- Protective features: *'What stops you from ending your life?'*
- Risk to others: *'Would you or have you thought about harming anyone else?"*

Past medical history: Any history of a mood or eating disorder, e.g. weight loss, excessive dieting, binge eating, laxative abuse

Family history – including psychiatric disease or suicide

Drug history – including illicit psychoactive substances, e.g. cocaine, cannabis, anabolic steroids

Social history – who do they live with, enquire about relationships with family, friends and partner. Any financial difficulties or problems at work/college? What is their support network?

Management:

1. Tell patient that you can advise the coach that they are not selectable for competition due to medical reasons, and you don't need to break confidentiality if they don't want you to explain the precise reasons
2. If high risk on suicide screening, the patient must be evaluated for safety with a full mental health evaluation
3. If patient admits to an overdose, then depending on substance and amount will require admission for observations, bloods and monitoring:
   a. Bloods for paracetamol and salicylate level and urine toxicology, FBC, U&E, LFTs, glucose, clotting and an arterial blood gas for acid-base disturbance
   b. ECG (prolonged PR and QRS with tricyclic antidepressants, prolonged QT with quinine)
   c. Possible trial of antidote where toxic agent known, e.g. N-acetylcysteine (NAC) in paracetamol, flumazenil for benzodiazepines
4. Addressing low mood
   a. Referral to a psychologist for psychotherapy, e.g. CBT to address low mood and anxiety
   b. Liaise with GP regarding consideration of SSRI
   c. May benefit from formal psychiatric referral and assessment for continuity of care, especially if suicide risk moderate to high
5. Offer to discuss with family or anyone in their support network and potentially arrange for early return home from tournament
6. Signpost to resources, e.g. Samaritans

MEMORY LOSS

"You are a GP with specialist interest in sports medicine. A 44-year-old retired professional rugby player comes to see you with his wife at her insistence. He says he has been struggling with his memory recently and his wife says she has noticed changes in his behaviour. He said he has got lost driving his car to local familiar locations such as the supermarket, a journey he normally makes one a week. His wife said he has left the stove on twice. He has also become more irritable and frustrated, snapping at this family more often than usual. He had a successful career playing elite rugby as a prop, suffering multiple head injuries during his career. He retired 2 years ago and now works as a rugby coach. He is concerned he has dementia due to the head injuries he sustained in the past, similar to cases he has seen in the news recently. Please take a history and explain your investigations and management plan."

History:

- Duration and onset of symptoms – insidious or sudden change?
- Ask for specific examples of confusion or memory loss – does he forget people, time of day, disorientated in familiar places
- Quality of long-term vs short-term memory – ask to recall remote and recent events
- Any problems in concentration, personal hygiene, emotions
- Detailed history of head injuries during career
- Any seizures, vascular symptoms, e.g. diplopia, vertigo, any neurological symptoms, e.g. ataxia, tremor or any other physical symptoms or evidence of a movement disorder e.g. tremor
- Degree of insight patient has into the symptoms
- Screen for underlying mood disorder – anhedonia, poor appetite, sleep disturbance
- Any hallucinations

Past medical history: Vascular risk factors

Family history: Any history of early-onset dementia (<60 years), Alzheimer's

Drug history: Any sedatives or significant alcohol history?

Social: Work demands, family, driving, risk assessment, i.e. cooking, heating

Ascertain detailed collateral history from wife regarding premorbid temperament, behaviour and understand the patient and wife's ideas, concerns and expectations.

Differential diagnosis:

- Medical cause – hypothyroidism, vitamin B12 deficiency, infection (viral encephalitis, prion disease), metabolic, e.g. kidney, failure, neoplastic, e.g. brain metastases, vascular, i.e. stroke, medications
- Early-onset dementia
  - Vascular
  - Alzheimer's
  - Dementia with Lewy bodies
  - Alcoholic dementia
  - Frontotemporal lobar degeneration
- Chronic traumatic encephalopathy (CTE)
- Mood disorder – depression, psychosis

Examination:

- Full examination of cardiovascular, respiratory and gastrointestinal system. Assess for carotid bruit and peripheral arterial disease which may indicate vascular cause. Neurological examination: Assess for extrapyramidal signs including tremor, bradycardia and rigidity, focal neurology indicating stroke or a space-occupying lesion

Investigations:

- Dementia screening tool, e.g. Montreal Cognitive Assessment (MoCA): Score > 26 considered normal
- Blood tests: FBC, U&E, LFT, thyroid function tests, triglycerides, cholesterol, HbA1c, erythrocyte sedimentation rate (ESR), vitamin B12, folate and ferritin, treponema pallidum
- Consider structural imaging, e.g. MRI head, to rule out reversible causes such as space-occupying lesion

Management:

- Investigations as above
- Specialist referral to neurologist or specialist memory clinic for further assessment, investigation and diagnostic dementia subtyping. This may include lumbar puncture (to rule out infection and assess for tau and amyloid-beta), single-photon emission computerised tomography (SPECT) or positron emission tomography (PET) scan

- Risk assessment including safety at home and discuss plan with wife +/− involve occupational therapy. Ensure no suicide risk. Develop a care and support plan and agree this with the patient and wife – provide written plan and date for review
- Consider treatment for comorbid mood disorders such as anxiety and/or depression
- Discuss with patient that at this stage you are unable to give a definitive diagnosis but that the investigations and referral to neurologist will be able to rule out simple causes and aid in diagnosis. With regards to their concern of CTE, explain there is no current consensus of clinical criteria to diagnose CTE and generally, it is diagnosed once other causes are ruled out
- Arrange follow-up

REFERENCES

1. Mountjoy M, et al. The IOC consensus statement: Beyond the female athlete triad–relative energy deficiency in sport (RED-S). *Br J Sports Med.* 2014: 491–7.
2. Morgan JF, Reid F, Lacey JH. The SCOFF questionnaire: A new screening tool for eating disorders. *West J Med.* 2000;172(3):164–5.
3. Mountjoy M, et al. IOC consensus statement on relative energy deficiency in sport (RED-S): 2018 update. *Br J Sports Med.* 2018:687–97.
4. Ackerman KE, et al. Oestrogen replacement improves bone mineral density in oligo-amenorrhoeic athletes: A randomised clinical trial. *Br J Sports Med.* 2019;53(4):229–36.
5. Griffin SA, Walsted ES, Hull JH. Breathless athlete: Exercise-induced laryngeal obstruction. *Br J Sports Med.* 2018:1211–12.
6. Dickinson JW, Hull JH. *Complete Guide to Respiratory Care in Athletes.* Routledge; 2020.
7. Gouttebarge V, et al. International Olympic Committee (IOC) Sport Mental Health Assessment Tool 1 (SMHAT-1) and Sport Mental Health Recognition Tool 1 (SMHRT-1): Towards better support of athletes' mental health. *Br J Sports Med.* 2021;55(1):30–7.
8. Gouttebarge V, Goedhart E, Kerkhoffs G. Empowering the health of retired professional footballers: The systematic development of an after career consultation and its feasibility. *BMJ Open Sport Exerc Med.* 2018;4(1):e000466.

INTRODUCTION

Previous communication stations in sport and exercise medicine objective structured clinical examinations (OSCEs) have focussed on clinical management for some of the commonly encountered conditions in sport and exercise medicine, including knowledge of a structured rehabilitation programme. As outlined in Chapter 1, for stations requiring an outline of a rehabilitation schedule, you should have a systematic approach outlining the different stages of rehabilitation with appropriate specific exercises at each stage. Often the patient will push you for an exact timescale which in practice is rarely accurate, but approximate timeframes can be suggested depending on the patient's progression. Present a balanced view of all the options if there is equivocal evidence of the long-term prognosis of different management options. If the patient is elite, then consider the wider management including psychological support and involvement of the multidisciplinary team (MDT). If it is a paediatric patient, then liaising with the school or coach and parents is necessary.

CLINICAL CASES

ANTERIOR CRUCIATE LIGAMENT (ACL) TEAR MANAGEMENT ADVICE

"John is a 28-year-old lacrosse player who sustained an isolated ACL tear 2 weeks ago. He has never had a lower limb injury or intervention before. He has come to ask some questions about potential management options."

Information gathering

- Establish current sporting level and his short- and long-term goals – a return to high performance cutting sports may influence advice
- Ascertain current level of knowledge of treatment options

- Establish the injury status of the supporting structures, e.g. meniscus, collaterals, any mechanical symptoms or giving way?
- Any previous injuries – is this a first-time ACL tear?
- Any previous treatment or surgery?

Information giving

- Operative and non-operative treatments are both acceptable treatment options for ACL injury
- Prior to a treatment decision being made, all patients should be offered supervised rehabilitation for at least 5 weeks consisting of strengthening and neuromuscular exercises which have been shown to improve quality of life and function (1). Patients can start rehabilitation when near full range of movement (ROM), minimal effusion and no quadriceps lag
- Evidence base:
  - Frobell showed rehabilitation plus early surgery not more beneficial than trial of rehabilitation first with the option of surgery at a later date (2) (Note: Patients with Grade 3 medial collateral ligament (MCL)/Lateral collateral ligament (LCL)/Posterior cruciate ligament (PCL), complex meniscal tears and full-thickness cartilage lesions were excluded from this study – see referral for surgery below)
  - Reijman showed that early reconstruction had improved symptoms and knee function (measured using the International Knee Documentation Committee score) vs rehabilitation with elective delayed reconstruction, but the study concluded it is unclear if there was any clinically significant difference (3)
- High risk of re-injury after ACL reconstruction
  - Risk of second ACL reinjury rate is 15% in athletes after ACL reconstruction (ipsilateral reinjury rate of 7% and contralateral

DOI: 10.1201/9781003163701-15

injury rate of 8%). Secondary injury rates for athletes <25 years is even higher at 21% (4)

- Risk of second ACL injury after ACL reconstruction is 18% in professional footballers (5)
  - Highest risk in first 9 months after injury
- Development of osteoarthritis (OA) after ACL tear is multifactorial, and evidence is inconclusive whether either treatment option reduces incidence of future OA
- Risks of surgery:
  - Procedure: Bleeding, pain, infection, deep vein thrombosis (DVT), stiffness
  - Graft failure (<1/10), patellofemoral joint (PFJ) pain if patellar graft
- Outline rehabilitation protocol and expected length of time to return to play (RTP; on average 6–9 months) (see Chapter 8)
- No difference in 2-year outcome measures after ACL repair if in an accelerated vs standard rehabilitation programme (6)
- Prognosis for RTP:
  - Rehabilitation is criteria-driven with progression to each stage determined by a battery of tests assessing clinical and functional progress
  - 65% recreational vs 83% professional athletes will return to pre-injury level of sport following surgery (7)
  - Regardless of treatment, injured knee has a 4.2× greater chance of developing OA compared to controls in 10 years (8)

Referral for surgery if:

- Instability in desired activity despite optimal rehabilitation
- If associated injury requiring surgery, e.g. bucket handle meniscal tear
- In active patients wishing to return to jumping, cutting and pivoting sports, operative treatment considered preferred option to maintain athletic participation in medium to long term (1–5+ years). In these patients, return to these types of sports without surgery may place the knee at risk of secondary injury to the meniscus or cartilage

Paediatric considerations (9)

- Determine skeletal age and likely further growth e.g. bone age from left-hand X-ray, parental height, Tanner stage – risk to physes if still open
- Techniques include transphyseal, physeal sparing and partial transphyseal
- Patellar tendon graft may damage tibial tubercle

- Conservative management is first line if skeletally immature and no associated injuries or major instability
- Risks of reconstruction: Growth disturbance (2%), secondary ACL rupture (25%–15% either side), 15% risk of graft rupture, knee stiffness, infection

Reach a shared decision based on patient's presentation, goals and presentation after explanation given of all of the options.

BONE STRESS INJURY (BSI)

"A 28-year-old international-level triple jumper has sustained a stress fracture of the calcaneum diagnosed on MRI. They are 2 months out from an Olympic qualifying competition. Please discuss the diagnosis and management plan with the athlete."

Information gathering

- Establish their understanding of a BSI and their expectations and goals from the outset
- Determine any reversible risk factors, especially lifestyle factors, e.g. nutritional and any recent changes in training load, surface or footwear (Table 12.1)
- Establish the location of fracture and severity – in this case, it is a low-risk location (Table 12.2). A high-risk location would require early surgical referral and possible non-weight bearing (NWB) pathway due to possibility of non or malunion or avascular necrosis (AVN). MRI may give an indication as to the grade of an early stress fracture which will also give some guidance on prognosis for RTP

Information giving and communicate plan

- Explain diagnosis and any probable risk factors
- Explain further investigations if required, e.g. bloods including bone profile and vitamin D, DEXA
- Explain management is milestone-driven, not determined by arbitrary time points
- Explain management plan:
  - Period of relative offloading with activity modification and relative rest +/− crutch or Aircast® boot, especially if pain when walking or rest pain
  - Analgesia (not non-steroidal anti-inflammatories [NSAIDs] as can impair bony healing)
  - Address underlying cause, e.g. education regarding training load progression not to exceed >10% per week

Table 12.1 Bone and load-related risk factors for developing a bone stress injury

Abnormal load, normal bone	Abnormal bone, normal load
Biomechanical	Low energy availability
• Leg length discrepancy	• Dietary evaluation
• Pes cavus	• Oligomenorrhoea
Training factors	• Current or previous ED
• Load – frequency, duration	Deficient in calcium or vitamin D
Playing surface	Coeliac disease
Footwear	History of corticosteroid use

ED, eating disorder.

- Optimise lifestyle measures, e.g. Stop smoking, dietary advice if under-fuelling and including vitamin D supplementation if insufficient or deficient
- Maintain ROM and cardiovascular (CV) fitness – swim, cycle, upper body strength and trunk stability
- Graded rehabilitation programme – tailor this to the injury
- Return to play governed by clinical assessment of pain, strength and ROM
  - In an elite setting, this will be daily assessment with involvement of MDT
- Address psychological aspects and involve MDT including coach, dietician, psychologist. Encourage athlete to attend team training sessions and meetings

Return to play after a bone stress injury

"The athlete has completed their graduated RCT protocol within 6 weeks and they want you to medically clear them for competition – what do you advise?"

- RTP should ideally be when strength, ROM and proprioception is equal to the uninjured side and successful completion of rehabilitation programme with minimal pain
- RTP is a balance between athlete's desire to compete and the possible risk of complications including delayed or non-union and further injury
- Liaise with the MDT and athlete together to evaluate their specific situation and make a shared decision

Top tips

- Understand the difference in treatment for low and high-risk stress fractures
- Ask questions to determine risk factors including training load, nutrition and biomechanics
- RTP decisions require shared decision making with frequent MDT discussion and clinical assessment
- Show empathy and be willing to work with athlete towards their aims. Some may wish to compete despite known further injury risk

Table 12.2 List of high- and low-risk location bone stress injuries

High risk	Low risk
Superior margin femoral neck	Inferior margin femoral neck
Anterior cortex of tibia	Posterior cortex of tibia
Medial malleolus	Femoral shaft
Navicular	Calcaneus
Patellar	Pelvis
Proximal diaphysis 5th MT	Pubic ramus
Base 2nd MT	Fibula
Proximal 2nd–4th MT	Diaphysis 2nd–4th MT
Sesamoids	
→ **Early surgical referral**	

MT, metatarsal.

TENDINOPATHY REHABILITATION

"You are asked to see a 60-year-old gentleman who is a keen runner and cyclist and has recently been diagnosed with midportion Achilles tendinopathy. He has controlled hyperlipidaemia. He has come to see you today to discuss management and in particular rehabilitation exercises and prognosis. You are not required to do an examination or establish the diagnosis."

Information giving

1. General information giving
   - Tendinopathy is a common condition which occurs when a tendon is unable to adapt to the strain placed on it. This can lead to structural changes within the tendon and pain
   - Risk factors include age, gender, weight and medical conditions. e.g. DM or biomechanical errors. A sudden change in training load can also precipitate it
   - Prolonged rest is detrimental and the mainstay of management is a progressive loading programme
   - Treatment can involve painkillers, relative rest, stretching, exercise programme and adjuncts
2. Rehabilitation
   - Rehabilitation course is on average 3-6 months and 10-50% do not respond
   - Expect noticeable change in symptoms by 4 weeks
   - Four stage programme: Isometrics, isotonics, energy storage and sport specific. Also include gastrocnemius and soleus stretches.
   - Try not to do consecutive days heavy loading
   - Maintain pain diary throughout to monitor response to load: aim <4/10 on visual analogue scale (VIS) and no flare the following day: *'Work to a level of pain you are comfortable with'*
   - Isometric – 45 seconds holding a calf raise, 5 repetitions (perform seated if pain+) with body weight (BW) or weights

     Progress once pain <5/10, no morning stiffness, low pain on single leg calf raise

   - Isotonic (continue isometrics alongside)
     - Slow and heavy concentric and eccentric, e.g. calf raises 3 seconds up and 4 seconds down, 3 sets of 8 repetitions on alternate days (or 3×/week)
     - Strengthen soleus as well and kinetic chain, e.g. quadriceps and glutes
     - Avoid loading on consecutive days, at least initially
   - Energy storage (continue isotonics twice per week): Twice per week, e.g. double leg hop, forward and backwards hop, side to side, then single leg hop
   - Sport specific, e.g. return to running programme, jumping, ball drills, change of direction

     RTP when can do above without exacerbation of pain

3. Other – continue cycling to maintain CV fitness
4. Advice on training load: Do not increase by 10% per week, increase cadence, reduce stride length
5. Refer for biomechanical assessment +/− orthotics
6. Refractory cases – consider dry needling, glyceryl trinitrate (GTN), sclerosing therapies or, extra-corporal shock wave therapy
   - Cochrane review shows steroid injection has no long-term benefit (10)
7. Surgery potentially considered as a last resort. There is currently no randomised controlled trial (RCT) comparing surgical vs conservative management

HAMSTRING INJURY REHABILITATION

"You are a sport and exercise medicine registrar, and you receive a phone call from a GP who has just seen an 18-year-old athlete who has acutely strained their hamstring muscle. They do not have access to any imaging within the next 2 weeks. The GP would like advice on how to manage and rehabilitate the athlete as they are inexperienced with this presentation. The athlete is asking him when he can return to competition."

Information gathering

- What was the mechanism of injury and when did it happen?
- Is this their first presentation or do they have a history of hamstring muscle injury?
- Could they immediately weight bear
- What are the findings on examination – bruising, palpable defect, antalgic gait, strength. Do they have back pain or neurological symptoms?
- What is the patient's level of competition and goal, e.g. when is the next competition they wish to compete in?
- Any medical conditions or drug history
- Occupation

Information giving

Rehabilitation progression is criteria-dependent, not time-dependent so you cannot give an exact timescale for return to play. However, as a general rule of thumb, muscle injuries take on average 3 weeks, musculotendinous junction (MTJ) injuries take 6 weeks and any tendon involvement can take 9+ weeks. Poorer prognosis is also associated with inability to weight bear initially.

Rehabilitation is divided into stages – acute, conditioning, sport specific and return to play:

Acute phase
- Protect, optimal loading, ice, compression elevation (POLICE), analgesia
- Muscle activation 3–4×/day, low-grade pain free, e.g. prone knee bends
- Aim for pain-free walking and restore ROM
- Maintain CV fitness throughout, e.g. rowing, stationary cycle, stepper

Can progress to next stage when walking pain free and isometric pain free

Subacute phase
1. Muscle strengthening
   - Muscle strengthening of hamstrings 3 sets of 12 repetitions
     - E.g. Hip extension and abduction, TheraBand™ exercises,
     - Bridges
     - Single leg roll out on a Swiss ball
     - Nordic hamstring exercises (high eccentric element so only do this late in rehabilitation)
     - Deadlifts
     - Delay eccentric exercises until late, especially if tendon involvement
   - Muscle strengthening synergists, i.e. gluteus maximus, adductor magnus
     - Squat, deep lunge
   - Neuromuscular (NM) control – proprioceptive exercises on BOSU® ball

Progress when can perform the above pain free, with good form and no guarding

2. Functional exercises
   - Return to running programme
   - Sport-specific drills, e.g. fast feet
3. Maintain CV fitness throughout
4. Attend training and address risk factors, e.g. muscle weakness or imbalances

Progress to training when no minimal symptoms and return to running programme completed, full and pain-free ROM, able to perform Askling H-test

RTP phase

Return to play once completed one week of full training

Indications for referral to specialist:

- Inability to progress through rehabilitation programme due to pain or dysfunction
- Any back pain or neurological symptoms – is this an L5 radiculopathy?

OSGOOD-SCHLATTER DISEASE

"You have been referred a 12-year-old school child by his GP for persistent knee pain. He currently plays hockey, football and cricket for the school and county rugby and football. His symptoms have continued despite regular NSAIDs and some physiotherapy. His GP suspects it is Osgood-Schlatter disease and has told him it will go away with time. He has come to speak to you with his father today. Please take a history and explain what you would look for on examination, then explain your management plan to the patient."

Information gathering

History:

- Age of onset 12–15 years in males, 8–12 years in females M:F 4:1
- Clinical features: Pain and swelling over tibial tubercle (Sinding-Larsen-Johansson [SLJ] will be at inferior patella pole). Symptoms exacerbated during periods of growth and by jumping and running
- Level of sport played and which sports played
- Establish if likely to grow further – parental height, previous growth spurts
- Screen for red flags – swelling, night pain, weight loss
- Important in paediatrics to ensure not being pushed by family/school coach: *'Do you feel you are being made to do these sports?'*

Examination:

- Point tenderness and bony swelling over tibial tubercle
- Quadriceps tightness (restricted knee flexion)
- Pain on resisted knee extension
- May have biomechanical abnormalities, e.g. pes planus
- May have PFP problems if prolonged

Information giving

- Explain the diagnosis and educate the patient and parent that symptoms are likely to last several seasons and symptoms will be worse during periods of rapid growth. However it otherwise has an excellent prognosis as 95% self-limit
- If they press for investigations, explain that it is a clinical diagnosis, and using ionising

radiation, e.g. X-ray is reserved for if the diagnosis in doubt or the patient has persistent symptoms.

Management:

- Activity modification – common in children who do multiple sports frequently. Come to a shared decision with patient and family to potentially cut down number of aggravating activities and focus on a few favoured sports.
  - Involve school coaches and parents so everyone on board – written letter
- Analgesia – can include topical NSAIDs and ice over area after training or competition, and to limit oral NSAIDs for important training sessions or big competitions to reduce side effects.
- Quadriceps flexibility and strengthening programme – to reduce traction of tight muscle on tibial tuberosity
  - E.g. Shoulder bridges, squats
- Correct any biomechanical abnormalities – check footwear including school shoes
- Surgical review if skeletally mature and persistent and disabling symptoms

REFERENCES

1. Eitzen I, et al. A progressive 5-week exercise therapy program leads to significant improvement in knee function early after anterior cruciate ligament injury. *J Orthop Sports Phys Ther.* 2010;40(11):705–21.

2. Frobell RB, et al. A randomized trial of treatment for acute anterior cruciate ligament tears. *N Engl J Med.* 2010;2010:331–42. Massachusetts Medical Society: United States.

3. Reijman M, et al. Early surgical reconstruction versus rehabilitation with elective delayed reconstruction for patients with anterior cruciate ligament rupture: COMPARE randomised controlled trial. *BMJ.* 2021;372:n375.

4. Wiggins AJ, et al. Risk of secondary injury in younger athletes after anterior cruciate ligament reconstruction: A systematic review and meta-analysis. *Am J Sports Med.* 2016;44(7):1861–76.

5. Della Villa F, et al. High rate of second ACL injury following ACL reconstruction in male professional footballers: An updated longitudinal analysis from 118 players in the UEFA Elite Club Injury Study. *Br J Sports Med.* 2021.

6. Beynnon BD, et al. Rehabilitation after anterior cruciate ligament reconstruction: A prospective, randomized, double-blind comparison of programs administered over 2 different time intervals. *Am J Sports Med.* 2005. 33(3): p. 347–59.

7. Lai CCH, et al. Eighty-three per cent of elite athletes return to preinjury sport after anterior cruciate ligament reconstruction: A systematic review with meta-analysis of return to sport rates, graft rupture rates and performance outcomes. *Br J Sports Med.* 2018:128–38.

8. Poulsen E, et al. Knee osteoarthritis risk is increased 4–6 fold after knee injury – A systematic review and meta-analysis. *Br J Sports Med.* 2019:1454–63.

9. Ardern CL, et al. 2018 International Olympic Committee consensus statement on prevention, diagnosis and management of paediatric anterior cruciate ligament (ACL) injuries. *Br J Sports Med.* 2018;52(7):422–38.

10. Kearney RS, et al. Injection therapies for Achilles tendinopathy. *Cochrane Database Syst Rev.* 2015(5): CD010960.

13 Clinical communication and ethics

INTRODUCTION

Clinical communication and ethics are commonly assessed in sport and exercise medicine objective structured clinical examinations (OSCEs). This can range from challenging communication situations such as breaking bad news to dealing with an angry patient or a 'pushy parent'. Practice dealing with these scenarios with peers and develop strategies to effectively deal with them. These stations could also consist of teaching scenarios or demonstrating practical procedures and this chapter has presented a structured approach which can be adopted in order to deliver a fluid and well-organised performance. If you are given a preparatory station beforehand, use this time wisely to plan and take notes on what you will say.

CLINICAL CASES

BREAKING BAD NEWS

"An 18-year-old gymnast presented 3 weeks ago with unilateral swelling above his knee. An X-ray was performed, and he has come to see you today with the results. X-rays show an abnormality arising from the bone with appearances in keeping with osteosarcoma. Please discuss with the patient."

"A 65-year-old male presented to you last month with lower back pain after recently taking up golf. You arranged a magnetic resonance imaging (MRI) scan of his lumbar spine which has shown multiple enhancing lesions consistent with bone metastases. There is no spinal cord compression. He is here to discuss the results of the scan."

Have a strategy for these type of stations and react appropriately to how they respond, e.g. if they start crying, pause and wait for them to finish before you go on. Despite being under time pressure, do not plough in immediately with the diagnosis, but work up to that moment by first building rapport and finding out what information they already know. Avoid the use of euphemisms or medical jargon.

Information gathering

1. Opening the conversation
   - Introduce yourself and ensure it is the correct patient
   - Ensure quiet room without interruptions
   - Ask if the patient is accompanied by anyone today and would they like them to sit in
   - Start with an open question. E.g. *'How have you been since I last saw you?'* Ask about other symptoms, e.g. weight loss, night sweats, shortness of breath (SOB)
   - Establish what the patient already knows or is expecting from this consultation, e.g. were differential diagnoses previously explored?
   - Ask them what they think the problem might be

Information giving

2. Breaking the news
   - Give a warning shot, e.g. *'You are here today to discuss the results of the scan, I'm afraid I have bad news'*. After this, leave a pause and see how the patient reacts.
   - Using simple language, explain the diagnosis: *'The scans show you have bone cancer'*
   - Deliver information in chunks and leave pauses after each bit of information
   - When timing is right, acknowledge this must be a big shock. Reassure that there are specialist centres to manage this illness with well-established treatments
   - Ask him if he wants to discuss the diagnosis in more detail
   - Recognise and respond to emotions with empathy, e.g. *'I'm really sorry to give you this news'*. If they respond with anger, acknowledge this and respond appropriately

DOI: 10.1201/9781003163701-16

- Do not mislead regarding prognosis
- Do not deliver a lot of information if the patient is upset or crying. Pause and give the patient a tissue and ask if it is OK to go on

3. Making a plan
- Set out next steps, e.g. arranging further investigations urgently, referring urgently to tertiary sarcoma team and will liaise regarding further urgent investigations, e.g. MRI, chest X-ray (CXR), bloods
- They may want to know treatment options, if you are not an expert, do not give false information: *'Treatment may involve chemotherapy or surgery, but the specialists will explain in more detail with you'*.
- Enquire about support, e.g. friends and family
- State you will inform and liaise with their GP
- Offer written information leaflets, signpost to websites and ensure they have your contact number
- Safety net at the end with information regarding red flag symptoms e.g. spinal cord compression

Common pitfalls:
- Not recognising when to be silent
- Giving too much information too quickly
- Misleading the patient, e.g. regarding prognosis

CONCUSSION

"A 17-year-old female rugby player sustained a head injury yesterday whilst going in for a tackle during a county-level match. She was immediately removed due to dizziness and headache. Today she comes to see you with her father as her coach said she needs clearance from the doctor before she can play in the cup final in one week. She is the top try scorer on the team. Her father is particularly unhappy as the physiotherapist has said that she should not play in a week. Please discuss the diagnosis and management plan with her and her father."

A concussion is a mild traumatic brain injury and refers to a clinical syndrome normally following head trauma. You should have knowledge of the return to play (RTP) guidelines for adults and under 19s and also know the difference in the standard versus enhanced return to play protocol. These scenarios may also focus around dealing with an imbalance in expectations between player and protocol such that the aim of the station may not be delivering the precise RTP protocol, but managing the player/parent's expectations and using careful communication and negotiation skills.

Information gathering

- Establish their understanding of concussion and their expectations
- Determine if she currently has any symptoms
- Find out if she has a history of prior concussion, how many episodes and how long ago
- Establish any past medical history, drug history and current education and sporting level played
- If father or player become pushy or angry at any point, acknowledge that it is frustrating for them and that it's clear they really want to play

Information giving

- Explanation of concussion as a type of traumatic brain injury
- Explain risks of early RTP following concussion:
  - Second impact syndrome
  - Post-concussive syndrome
  - 3× increased risk of second concussion and musculoskeletal injury
  - Poor performance
  - Growing evidence linking concussion to Chronic traumatic encephalopathy
- Research shows that the paediatric/adolescent brain and females require longer rest
- Briefly safety net with explanation of red flags
- Explain that national guidelines dictate return to play timeframes, and you are unable to give clearance prior to or deviate from this

Communicate plan – Standard return to play protocol in under 19s

Six stage graduated return to play (Table 13.1) (1). If symptoms return at any point, rest for 48 hours and drop back to the previous stage:

Stage 1: Initial rest 14 days (24–48 hours complete rest)
- 24–48 hours complete rest followed by continuation of initial rest period of 14 days total
- Complete rest: Complete physical and mental rest required including time off school (liaise with school if necessary)
- Do not leave alone for first 48 hours
- Minimal screen time
- Minimal gaming
- No exercise
- Advice against driving
- No alcohol
- No prescription or non-prescription drug including sedatives, non-steroidal anti-inflammatories (NSAIDs), aspirin without medical supervision
- After complete rest period to reintroduce normal activities of daily living

Table 13.1 Six stage standard and enhanced return to play protocol

	Stage 1	Stage 2	Stage 3	Stage 4	Stage 5	Stage 6 earliest RTP
Standard adult	14 days	24 hours	24 hours	24 hours	24 hours	Day 19
Standard U17–19	14 days	48 hours	48 hours	48 hours	48 hours	Day 23
Enhanced adult	24 hours	24 hours	24 hours	24 hours	24 hours	Day 6
Enhanced U17–19	7 days	24 hours	24 hours	24 hours	24 hours	Day 12

U17–19, under 17–19 years of age; RTP, return to play.

Clearance by doctor recommended prior to Stage 2

Stage 2 – Light exercise   48 hours
- Walking, light jogging, swimming, stationary cycling

Stage 3 – Sport specific   48 hours
- Running drills, adding movement but no impact activities

Stage 4 – Non-contact training   48 hours
- Passing drills, change of direction, resistance training can begin

→*Doctor review prior to Stage 5*

Stage 5 – Full contact practice   48 hours
- Normal training activities

Stage 6 – RTP

Liaise with coach regarding correct tackle techniques and address any risky playing behaviours.

Closing

- Check understanding and provide written information or signpost to website
- Build rapport with patient and parent and highlight clear guidelines if they are pushing for earlier return to play
- If patient or parent becomes angry, demanding a faster return to play, explain that guidelines cannot be reduced, especially in paediatric population. Offer a second opinion if necessary. Stress that your priority is to protect the health of the player
- Liaise with school and coach to ensure a co-ordinated management and prevention approach
- Consider referral to a neurologist if ongoing symptoms or multiple concussions

Note: Athletes aged 16 and under cannot follow an enhanced protocol and must adhere to the standard U17-19 protocol, i.e. earliest RTP is day 23.

At the time of writing, complete rest is initially advocated for adolescents with concussion, however one RCT has found early treatment with sub-symptom threshold aerobic exercise may speed recovery compared vs placebo stretching (2).

PATIENT SEEKING PASSIVE TREATMENT

"A 15-year-old female footballer comes to see you before an important cup match this afternoon. She says that she sprained her ankle yesterday during training, but didn't make a big deal of it and played on, because she really wants to play today. Today it is quite sore and she has asked you if you can give her an injection of local anaesthetic into the ankle to reduce the pain during the match. She says her father told her an injection will help her play this afternoon."

Information gathering

- Take a brief history to understand the mechanism of injury (MOI)
- Ask about current symptoms, range of movement (ROM) and strength
- Ask about nature of the game this afternoon and upcoming matches over the season
- Any previous injury to that ankle and/or treatment
- Enquire where she has read or heard about therapeutic injections. If she mentions that someone else, e.g. coach, another player or family member, has suggested she get an injection, explore this a little. How does *she* feel about getting an injection? Is there anything else that she is being asked to do? (Try to avoid leading questions if possible)
- Ask if you can examine her in order to rule out other more serious diagnoses and to screen for Ottawa ankle criteria to ensure she does not need X-rays

Information giving

- Assuming that the examination is satisfactory and there is no gross instability or loss of function, explain that the mainstay of management should be conservative and during this acute period this would include ice, strapping to reduce excessive ROM, elevation and analgesia. There are several things they can do now to manage her pain so that she can potentially play this afternoon, and then they can agree a longer-term plan for formal rehabilitation

- Explain that a 'short-term fix' isn't the best option – the risk of anaesthetising the ankle joint to enable her to play will be to mask the pain and potentially cause a more serious injury at a time when her strength and proprioception may be reduced
  - E.g. 70% of ankle osteoarthritis is secondary to a previous injury, so playing on an injured ankle may cause other longer-term issues
- Acknowledge and address the stress that she may be under and explore further if she is being coerced by her parent into more aggressive treatment. Offer to hold a meeting with the coach, physiotherapist, player (and father if she wants) to explain your medical advice on managing the injury, to take the onus off the player
- Reassure the player that she can come to you at any time if she has an illness, injury or concern in absolute confidence
- If in the exploration of the history there are warnings signs of controlling behaviour, then this should prompt a possible referral to the safeguarding lead for the organisation

Closing

- Reassure the patient that there are a lot of treatments you can offer to help her with symptoms, but in your professional opinion, you would not recommend an injection
- Offer to hold a team meeting to arrange a suitable rehabilitation plan going forward
- Address any additional psychological or social pressures the young athlete may be experiencing within the team and offer to have a discussion with her parent if she would like you to explain the situation
- Have a low threshold to explore underlying issues and appropriate onwards referral if necessary

BACK PAIN WITH NORMAL LUMBAR MRI

"You are due to see Mrs Jones for a follow-up appointment in a sport and exercise medicine clinic. She is a 67-year-old woman who was referred by her GP for a 12-month history of lower back pain. Mrs Jones has already seen the spinal team, two different physiotherapists and also a chiropractor for her chronic back pain. She is frustrated as they have all said there is 'nothing wrong' with her back. She has a background of irritable bowel syndrome and depression. At the moment she struggles to go on long walks like she used to and finding a comfortable sleeping position at night is difficult due to her pain.

On your initial assessment there were no red flag signs or neurological signs. Due to the chronicity of the symptoms, an MRI spine was performed to rule out serious underlying pathology. MRI demonstrates some degenerative osteophytes and loss of disc height but there are no other abnormalities. She has come today to discuss the scan results and ongoing management."

It is important to remember that in these stations where there is no 'organic pathology', the patient's symptoms may be debilitating and should be acknowledged. It is important to try and establish a rapport from the beginning in order to have a constructive discussion afterwards about management and prognosis. There are several management options to offer someone which should be tailored to the individual. 'Yellow flags' are psychosocial factors associated with an increased likelihood of chronic back pain and disability requiring a holistic approach to management addressing all biopsychosocial needs.

Yellow flags

- A negative attitude that back pain is harmful or potentially severely disabling
- Fear avoidance behaviour and reduced activity levels
- An expectation that passive, rather than active, treatment will be beneficial
- A tendency to depression, low morale and social withdrawal
- Social or financial problems

Information gathering

- Establish that she is here to discuss the results of her scan today
- Ask if there has been any change in her symptoms
- Ask how her symptoms are currently affecting her and how they impact her life. Let her speak without interrupting. If she expresses frustration at not being given a diagnosis, listen patiently to her
- Show genuine empathy for how her back pain is negatively affecting her life
- Set the agenda: *'Today we will discuss the scan results and then we will go through a plan together about how to manage your symptoms'*

Information giving

- Explain that the scan was done in order to rule out any sinister or reversible causes of her back pain and that reassuringly there are no abnormal structural features.
- Explain that pain is the body's reaction to a damaging stimulus. Sometimes the brain's

interpretation of this stimulus goes wrong and it keeps sending out pain signals with no obvious cause

- Reassure the patient that her symptoms are clearly real, despite there being no abnormalities on the scan, and that there are a number of different measures that you can put into place to address her symptoms which have been proven to help the quality of life in patients with chronic back pain
- Ask if there are any particular features that she finds debilitating and what her priorities are – this will help you individualise and tailor her management
- Explain the mainstay of management is multimodal to address her pain, her physical functioning and her psychological wellbeing and sleep. These can include:
  - Graded exercise therapy within pain limits which strengthen core and abdominal muscles. Explain that 'hurt doesn't mean harm'
  - Sensible analgesia plan with avoidance of opioids, but using a short course NSAIDs and heat and or ice at times of particularly troublesome symptoms may provide benefit
  - Sleep hygiene advice
  - Referral for psychological informed physiotherapy and/or cognitive therapy
  - If appropriate, refer to occupational therapy to help adapt daily activities
  - Liaise with GP about reviewing depression and whether SSRIs can be optimised
  - The StarT Back screening tool (3) can be used to stratify into low, medium and high-risk groups which allows targeted intervention
  - Offer leaflets and signpost to helpful websites on chronic lower back pain
  - Chronic pain team referral can be considered for those not responding to treatment as above which may include a pain education session, consideration of therapeutic injection, medication review and psychological therapies
  - Finish the consultation by summarising the plan, ask if she has any questions and organising suitable follow-up

CONFLICT MANAGEMENT – THE ANGRY PATIENT

"George Smith, a 16-year-old boy, has attended the Accident and Emergency (A&E) Department with his mother after feeling pain in the back of his thigh whilst sprinting for the ball during a school football match. A FY2 doctor in A&E diagnosed him with a muscle strain and advised conservative management and to reattend if the pain persisted. He reattended 2 days later due to persistent pain and difficulty weight bearing and another junior doctor prescribed analgesia and discharged home without investigations. You are a specialist registrar reviewing George today in the Sport and Exercise Medicine (SEM) clinic with his mother after they paid privately for an X-ray which has shown a large avulsion of the tibial tuberosity. His mother is very angry about the missed diagnosis and wants to make a formal complaint."

This scenario is not testing your medical knowledge of the injury and whether previous assessment and treatment was correct or not, but your ability to deal with conflict and anger and communication. You should make yourself familiar with the complaints procedure in your local healthcare trust and nationally.

- Whether a patient or their family is justified in their anger, the task should be to provide good clinical care, acknowledge their concerns and provide a constructive solution to handling their complaint
- Make sure that you listen to their concerns and express regret for the experience they have had to date
- Avoid making judgmental comments about the health professionals they saw previously as this may reinforce their belief and/or undermine their trust in healthcare services
- Reassure that, in most cases, avulsions can be managed conservatively. Explain that you would like to do a full examination and potentially arrange further imaging. Explain the treatment pathway will consist of relative rest, analgesia and physiotherapy and that you will discuss with the surgical team regarding whether he is a candidate for surgery.
- Listening and explaining in simple terms what has happened and what are the options for addressing their concerns should diffuse the situation. If a patient or their family get increasingly angry, remain calm and do not get defensive
- Explain that should they wish to make a complaint, there is a formal complaints procedure in place which should be followed. In the United Kingdom (UK), typically, this would include:
  - First stage: Local resolution
  - Second stage: Parliamentary and Health Service Ombudsman
  - Third stage: Judicial review

Advise them that their complaint should be made within 12 months of the incident, and they should receive a written acknowledgement within a week, however, local timelines vary. Signposting them to the Patient Advice and Liaison Service (PALS) is a useful first port of call.

- You can apologise on behalf of the healthcare trust you are working for, even if you haven't done something wrong personally, and carefully explain the steps you will take to help them
- Carefully document in the notes the discussions that have taken place and notify the consultant at the earliest available opportunity. The consultant is also best placed to communicate with the two junior doctors who initially saw George and will need to be informed with accompanying accurate and detailed medical notes
- Finish the consultation by summarising the plan going forward, ask if they are happy with the new plan and ensure they have timely follow-up

TEACHING STATIONS

Teaching stations can commonly arise in any medical specialty OSCE as it is assessing a fundamental skill required of all clinicians. However, even if you do teach regularly, it is easy to miss marks for timed teaching stations if you have not practiced one previously. It is important to realise that you will not pick up all the marks for a perfect didactic lecture of your knowledge of the area being asked to teach. A significant proportion of the marks will be dedicated to your ability to communicate, teach, feedback to the learner and structure the station. It is useful to differentiate between whether you are teaching someone how to perform a skill versus teaching a topic more knowledge based, e.g. the anatomy of the hand. Often you will be given some time to plan the station so use this to your advantage. Drawing a quick anatomical drawing to refer to during the station may aid understanding. If asked to cover a large subject area or examination, then select only a portion of this to teach depending on the length of the station to give you enough time for introductions, feedback and a summary.

If teaching how to perform a skill and/or you have a longer session with time to prepare, ideally use the 4-stage approach (4). The 4-stage approach to the teaching of skills has been adopted by the Advanced Life Support Group (ALSG) and Resuscitation Council (RC) (UK) and allows for repetition of the teaching component whilst allowing time for practice.

1. **Demonstration:** The teacher performs the skill in real time without comment. This step is taken to provide a benchmark
2. **Deconstruction:** The teacher performs every step slowly with an added explanation. The skill should be divided into smaller subsections

3. **Comprehension:** The student describes every step of the skill whereupon the teacher performs on instruction. The description and execution do not occur simultaneously
4. **Execution:** The student simultaneously narrates and executes step by step. At this stage, you can provide feedback as they are performing the skill or give feedback at the end

If the OSCE station is an ad hoc teaching opportunity, the 4-stage approach may not be practical due to time constraints. In this setting, it is more reasonable to use the following structure:

Setting the scene
- Introductions
- State what you will cover

Establish prior experience
- Level of baseline knowledge
- What is their objective

Talk through the procedure (led by learner):
- Ideally show, then show with commentary (you then them), then let them practice

Tips and tricks (provided by trainer)

Undertake procedure (with direct supervision)

Post-procedure feedback

"You are an SEM registrar and have been asked to give a 10-minute teaching session to a medical student on how to examine the foot and ankle."

Depending on the length of the station, you may wish to focus on a portion of the examination, e.g. observation, palpation and movement.

Setting the scene
- Introduce yourself and your role
- Ascertain the grade of the student
- State what you will aim to cover in the teaching station

Establish prior experience
- Ascertain the level of baseline knowledge of the student
- Find out what their objective is, e.g. learn for an OSCE, learn for orthopaedic rotation

Talk through the examination: Outline fundamental approach: Look, feel, move, special tests

Tips and tricks (provided by trainer): Exposure, positioning of patient

Undertake examination
- Show what you are looking for in observation including gait assessment
- Palpate the major structures of the foot and ankle and assess active and passive power. Provide commentary whilst doing so
- Next, allow the student to practice what you have just done and ask them to comment on what they are assessing for
- Provide real time feedback with practical tips on their technique

Post-procedure feedback
- Ask if any questions
- Summarise what you have covered and how it will be useful, e.g. 'Today we have covered observation, palpation and movement of the foot and ankle. This will help you in your examination on your orthopaedic placement'
- Schedule a follow-up, e.g. to go over special tests and recap learning from this session
- Signpost to resources

"You have been asked to demonstrate to a more junior colleague on the ward how to aspirate a knee effusion. You need to consent the patient and then demonstrate on the dummy provided."

Setting the scene
- Introduce yourself and your role
- Ascertain the grade of the junior doctor and if performed before

Establish Prior experience
- Ascertain the level of baseline knowledge and experience, e.g. other joint injections
- Find out what their objective is, e.g. formative or summative

Talk through the procedure (led by learner)
- Consent from patient and talk through consent process
- Discuss indications, contraindications, equipment required, interpretation of results
- Approach, e.g. medial retropatellar vs superolateral

Tips and tricks (provided by trainer)
- Specific information about the approach used
- Draw a diagram if useful

Undertake procedure (with direct supervision)
- If on a dummy, ideally show, then show with commentary (you then them), then let them practice
- Correct them if required when they practice
- Provide positive feedback as they practice

Post-procedure feedback
- Ask if any questions
- Signpost to resources, e.g. simulation courses

JOINT ASPIRATION AND INJECTION

It is unlikely that you will be required to perform an ultrasound-guided aspiration or injection of a joint, but it is possible you could be asked to perform aspiration or injection on a dummy using anatomical landmarks of some of the common joint injections. You should have knowledge of the indications and contraindications for injection,

the process of consent and be able to competently perform the procedure and provide aftercare advice.

"You have been referred a patient with confirmed carpal tunnel syndrome refractory to treatment. Please could you consent the patient for, and show how you would perform a therapeutic steroid injection of the carpal tunnel."

"You have reviewed a young man with an atraumatic knee effusion. You have been asked to consent the patient for a joint aspiration, perform the aspiration with the equipment provided and explain what investigations you would consider."

Diagnostic aspiration of the knee joint

1. Introduction and consent
   - Introduce yourself to the patient and confirm their name and date of birth
   - Confirm their understanding that they are to have some fluid removed from the knee to send off for analysis for the purposes of diagnosis
   - Explain aspiration may reduce the discomfort slightly
   - Briefly explain the procedure to the patient
   - Check if they have any absolute or relative contraindications:
     - Active infection
     - Broken skin
     - Low platelets or bleeding diatheses
     - Joint prosthesis
   - Explain the risks to the patient: Pain, bleeding, infection, damage to local structures, e.g. cartilage
   - Ask if they have any questions
2. Diagnostic aspiration
   - Set up equipment
     - Sterile procedure pack, betadine swabs, 20-mL syringe ×2, green needle (21g) ×2, cotton wool, plaster (if not allergic), lidocaine 1–2% (if using), sterile gloves, apron
   - Position patient (for medial retropatellar approach)
     - Place pillow under the knee (can also slightly internally rotate knee)
     - Palpate superior and inferior poles of patellar and locate the midpoint between these two locations
     - Palpate this midpoint just retropatellar for a soft space (medial glide of patella can sometimes accentuate) and mark point with the back of a needle cap

Note: A superolateral approach can be used, especially if there is a large knee effusion in the suprapatellar bursa. Have the knee in the extended position. Palpate the superior lateral aspect of the patella and mark a point 1 cm above and 1 cm lateral to this site. Aim the needle 45° towards the centre of the patella and directly slightly posteriorly and inferomedially into the knee joint.

- Aspiration
  - Wash hands and apply personal protective equipment (PPE) including plastic apron and sterile gloves
  - Place a green needle onto a 20-mL syringe
  - Clean the area with a sterile swab and leave to air dry
  - Using a no-touch technique, advance the needle as described aimed horizontally and slightly inferior underneath the patellar, aspirating as you advance. When syringe starts to fill with fluid, stop advancing and aspirate 20 mL of fluid
- Remove the needle and apply pressure with cotton wool. When haemostasis is achieved, apply a plaster if not allergic
- Closing
  - Transfer the fluid into sterile containers and send for microscopy, culture and sensitivities, cell count/cytology, crystal analysis and glucose. Also, arrange for appropriate blood tests if not already performed, e.g. full blood count (FBC), urea and electrolytes (U&E), C-reactive protein (CRP), erythrocyte sedimentation rate (ESR), urate
  - Document the consent and procedure
  - Provide aftercare advice: rest joint for 24–48 hours, safety net for signs of infection including swelling, pain, erythema, provide written leaflet and telephone number
  - Explain who will contact them for follow-up with results
  - Give patient an opportunity to ask questions

Therapeutic steroid injection of the carpal tunnel

1. Introduction and consent
   - Introduce yourself to the patient and confirm their name and date of birth
   - Confirm their understanding that they are here today to receive a steroid injection of the carpal tunnel.
   - Establish their understanding of the current situation
   - Explain the intended benefit is to provide temporary relief for her current symptoms +/– facilitate rehabilitation
   - Explore alternatives

Table 13.2 Risks associated with therapeutic corticosteroid injections

Risks	Rare
Local	• Anaphylaxis
• Pain or a flare in symptoms	• Tendon rupture
• Bleeding	• AVN
• Infection	• Nerve damage
• Lipodystrophy	
• Hypopigmentation	
Systemic	
• Flushing	
• Hyperglycaemia	
• Increase in BP	

AVN, avascular necrosis; BP, blood pressure.

- Briefly explain the procedure to the patient including the use of local anaesthetic and steroid
- Check if they have any absolute or relative contraindications
  - Active infection
  - Broken skin
  - Low platelets or bleeding diatheses
  - Allergy to lidocaine or steroid
  - Pregnancy
  - Poorly controlled type 2 diabetes mellitus (T2DM)
  - Breastfeeding
  - Menopausal
- Explain the risks to the patient (Table 13.2)
2. Joint injection
   - Set up equipment
     - Sterile procedure pack, betadine swabs, 2-mL syringe, green needle (21g) and blue needle (23g), vial of triamcinolone 10 mg, vial of lidocaine 1–2%, cotton wool, plaster (if not allergic), sterile gloves, apron
     - Wash hands and apply PPE including plastic apron and sterile gloves
     - Draw up triamcinolone using green needle into 2-mL syringe and make up the rest with lidocaine. Swap to blue needle which you will use to inject
3. Position patient
   - Place pillow under arm with palm facing up
   - Identify and mark the anatomy (Figure 13.1)
     - Find transverse crease of wrist
     - Find palmaris longus by asking them to oppose their thumb and little finger
     - Palpate radial and ulnar artery
   - Can mark injection site with the back of a needle cap - inject **ulnar** to palmaris

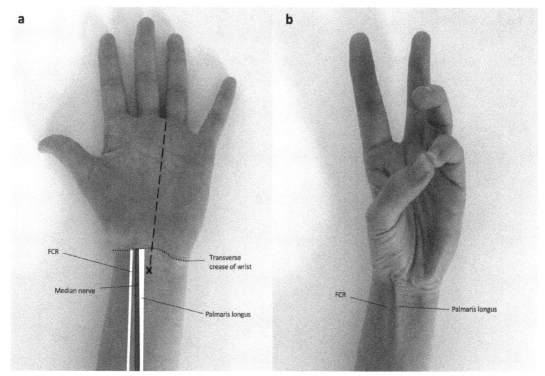

Figure 13.1 Anatomical landmarks for performing a therapeutic corticosteroid injection of the carpal tunnel. (a) Injection site (marked with an 'x') is 1 cm distal to the transverse crease of the wrist and on the ulnar side of the palmaris longus to avoid the median nerve, aiming towards the radial border of the ring finger. (b) To help identify anatomical landmarks prior to marking, ask the patient to oppose their thumb and little finger, which accentuates the palmaris longus in most people. FCR, flexor carpi radialis.

longus (median nerve is radial) approximately 1 cm down from transverse crease of the wrist, directing the needle 30° oblique under the transverse carpal ligament and aiming towards the radial border of the ring finger. Avoid obvious fine veins.

- Clean the area with a sterile swab and leave to air dry
- Advance needle as described above using a no-touch technique, aspirate to ensure not in a vessel and give as bolus. If resistance felt, do not proceed and attempt to readjust position of needle
- Remove the needle and apply pressure with cotton wool. When haemostasis achieved, apply plaster

4. Closing
- Document the consent and procedure
- Provide aftercare advice: Rest joint for 24–48 hours, safety net for signs of infection including swelling, pain, erythema, provide written leaflet and telephone number
- Give the patient an opportunity to ask questions

Anatomical landmarks and suggested injectate for other joints

As a general rule, use hydrophilic injectable steroids, e.g. hydrocortisone, for superficial injections to avoid the complication of lipoatrophy from lipophilic steroids, e.g. triamcinolone or methylprednisolone. A summary of suggested needle size and injectate is summarised in Table 13.3.

Ankle joint (anterior approach)

- Ankle in neutral position
- Palpate anterior joint line and identify extensor hallucis longus (EHL) and tibialis anterior. Safe entry point is between these two tendons approximately 1 cm below the anterior joint line (Figure 13.2). Direct the needle posteriorly
- Avoid dorsalis pedis artery which runs lateral to EHL

Glenohumeral joint (posterior approach)

- Have patient seated and ask to place hand on opposite leg (to internally rotate the shoulder)

Table 13.3 Suggested needle size, syringe and injectate for therapeutic corticosteroid injections of commonly injected joints

Site	Size needle	Size syringe	Injectate
Large joint, e.g. knee, ankle, glenohumeral joint	Green (21g) Ankle may require blue needle (23g)	5 mL	20–40 mg triamcinolone with the remaining made up of 1–2% lidocaine (max 3 mg/kg)
Subacromial bursa	Green (21g)	10 mL	20–40 mg triamcinolone + remaining lidocaine
Plantar fascia	Green (21g)	5 mL	20 mg triamcinolone + remaining lidocaine
Acromioclavicular joint	Orange needle (25g)	2 mL	1 mg triamcinolone + remaining lidocaine
Carpal tunnel	Blue needle (23g)	2 mL	10 mg triamcinolone + remaining lidocaine
De Quervain's tenosynovitis	Blue needle (23g)	2 mL	25 mg hydrocortisone + remaining lidocaine

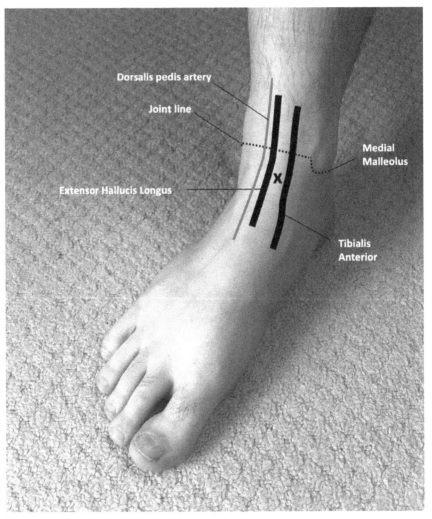

Figure 13.2 Anatomical landmarks for performing an ankle joint injection. Injection site is marked with an 'x' and is 1 cm distal to joint line and between tibialis anterior and extensor hallucis longus tendons.

- Palpate the posterior angle of the acromion with thumb and coracoid with the index finger and mark 1 cm below and 1 cm medial to the acromion landmark
- Needle entry will be at this point with direction towards the coracoid process

Subacromial bursa (posterior approach)

- As above but direct needle oblique and cranial aiming towards the acromioclavicular joint (ACJ)

De Quervain's tenosynovitis

- Flex thumb and ulnar deviate the wrist (Finkelstein's)
- Direct needle into sheath superficially, injecting distal to proximal

Elbow joint

- Have the patient seated with their elbow flexed at 45°
- Palpate and mark the landmarks of the lateral triangle which include the lateral epicondyle, radial head and lateral olecranon (Figure 13.3)
- This lateral approach will avoid the ulnar nerve
- Insert the needle at the centre of this triangle with the needle aimed towards the medial epicondyle

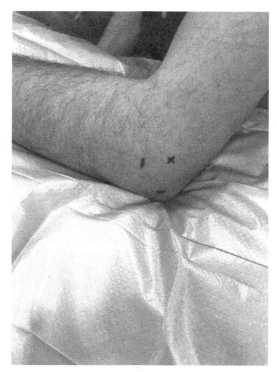

Figure 13.3 Anatomical landmarks for performing an elbow joint aspiration or injection. Landmarks of the lateral triangle have been marked including the lateral epicondyle (cross), radial head and lateral olecranon.

REFERENCES

1. McCrory P, et al. Consensus statement on concussion in sport: The 5(th) International Conference on Concussion in Sport, Berlin, October 2016. *Br J Sports Med*. 2017:838–47.
2. Leddy J, et al. Early targeted heart rate aerobic exercise versus placebo stretching for sport-related concussion in adolescents: a randomised controlled trial. *Lancet Child Adolesc Health*. 2021;30:S2352–4642.
3. Hay EM, et al. A randomised clinical trial of subgrouping and targeted treatment for low back pain compared with best current care. The STarT back trial study protocol. *BMC Musculoskelet Disord*. 2008;9:58.
4. Bullock I, et al. *Pocket Guide to Teaching for Clinical Instructors*. 2016, 3rd Edition, Wiley Blackwell.

14 Exercise medicine and public health

INTRODUCTION

Both public health and exercise prescription stations in chronic disease or special groups (e.g. pregnancy) have arisen in Sport and Exercise Medicine (SEM) objective structured clinical examinations (OSCEs). These stations are best tackled with a clear structure. Exercise prescription stations should be tailored according to the patient's preferences and barriers, which should be specifically explored. Motivational interviewing techniques are also useful to approach individuals who may be ambivalent about change. It is beyond the scope of this chapter to cover motivational interviewing techniques in detail, but it will cover some of the main points you should aim to cover in a 10-minute station.

PUBLIC HEALTH INTERVENTION

"You have been invited to be an advisor for a company looking to improve wellbeing and physical activity (PA) levels in their staff. Outline an initiative for a national company to encourage workers to be more active. The average worker works from home 2 days per week."

The best way to approach these type of stations is to break it down into different sections in order to structure your answer. This can be done in several ways but some suggestions include temporal, e.g. planning stage, implementation stage and evaluation phase, or to divide the proposed measures using a "ladder of interventions" as defined by the Nuffield Council on Bioethics [1] (Table 14.1).

Information gathering

- First, collect information on the number of workers, hours of PA per week (e.g. using the International Physical Activity Questionnaire [IPAQ]) and preferences and barriers, gender split, age split, potentially send out a survey
- Ensure inclusive and non-discriminatory
- Consider funding
- Consider local stakeholders, e.g. management, workforce, General Practitioners

- Define outcomes – short and long term using a 'logic model'
- Process evaluation of complex interventions: e.g. using the MRC guidance which focusses on implementation, mechanisms and context (2)
- Are there sufficient resources and staffing to deliver this? – action group, funding for questionnaires, time spent collating
- If appropriate, include a risk assessment. What will the procedure be if there is an adverse outcome, handling and storage of data as per General Data Protection Regulation (GDPR) guidance.

Intervention ladder

The interventions below are suggestions for designing a PA and wellbeing initiative for the company based on the intervention ladder framework. Depending on your information gathering phase you can tailor these interventions based on the needs of the company and staff.

Nudge 'Messaging'
- Education: Common messages: Send out weekly newsletters detailing the benefits of physical activity and simple lists of activities that you can undertake for free, e.g. walking, dancing
- Clearly outline the Chief Medical Officer (CMO) PA guidelines
- Create bike lanes around company buildings
- Brief line managers to introduce the discussion with mentees regarding wellbeing and activity
- Signpost to websites, e.g. Walk4life website (https://walk4life.info)
- Provide free pedometers

Shove 'Enabling'
- Healthier default policy, e.g. limit lifts to two people, so more people have to take the stairs
- Instigate cheaper healthy food options

DOI: 10.1201/9781003163701-17

Table 14.1 'Ladder of interventions' as defined by the Nuffield Council on Bioethics

Eliminate choice
Restrict choice
Guide choice by disincentives
Guide choice by incentives
Guide choice by changing the default policy
Enable choice
Provide information
Do nothing

- Organise company fitness challenge to encourage community or competition or group challenge – donate to charity?
- Provide bike-to-work scheme and vouchers
- Built environment changes – provide subsidised gym access
- Organise walking meetings
- Outline the need to spend commuting time when working from home on an active task
- Organise team building days with sporting activities, e.g. table tennis

Smack 'Penalise or make mandatory'
- Increase parking charges at the company
- Make compulsory breaks in meetings to take a walk
- Have a quota for steps/activity in appraisal meetings
- Managers to highlight to individuals who are not meeting current government guidelines

Summarise and closing
- Summarise your intervention plan based on your intervention ladder.
- Audit and review interventions at timely intervals with questionnaires to staff
- Undertake an evaluation of outcomes
- Arrange presentation to chief executive of results and next steps
- Disseminate findings to all stakeholders
- Publish and present outcomes

EXERCISE PRESCRIPTION

Exercise prescriptions stations should be divided into an information gathering section in which you explore the patient's goals, motivators and barriers, followed by delivering the prescription in a concise and tailored way. The Faculty of Sport and Exercise Medicine has written a clear and practical guide to exercise prescription [3] and Moving Medicine (www.movingmedicine.ac.uk) is also an excellent resource to utilise for healthcare professionals. There are also various motivational interviewing short courses that you can attend to put the techniques into practice.

Basic structure for an exercise prescription consultation
Overview:
- Use simple, open-ended questions
- Clarify and summarise what the patient has said during the consultation
- Ensure to check understanding throughout

Introduction:
- Establish the reason for attending or reason for referral and set the scene: *'I would like to take a few minutes today to discuss your physical activity if that's OK'*
- Start with open questioning techniques

Information gathering
- Establish their current and previous physical activity – intensity, frequency and duration
  - Physical activity, exercise or sport participation?
  - Domestic chores, e.g. gardening, hoovering
  - Physical activity related to occupation, e.g. lifting
- You may need to do a risk assessment regarding their suitability to start exercise (see below)
  - Current known cardiovascular, respiratory or metabolic **disease**
  - Any **symptoms** of cardiovascular, respiratory or metabolic disease
  - Any cardiovascular, respiratory or metabolic **risk factors**
  - Family history including sudden cardiac death (SCD)
  - Examination including height, weight, body mass index (BMI), waist circumference, heart sounds, pulse, blood pressure, urine dip, blood sugar
  - Use a Physical Activity Readiness Questionnaire (PAR-Q+) or equivalent validated questionnaire
  - Drug history, smoking and alcohol
- Find out the patient's **goals** (e.g. lose weight, walk to park with grandchildren), **preferred method** (e.g. group or individual activity, indoor or outdoor) and any **barriers** (childcare, financial, time) – this will help you tailor the prescription
  - Use reflective listening: *'It sounds like you've thought a lot about the way you want to make a change', 'It's clearly important to you to stay active for your family'*

- Calculate where in the 'Stages of Change' they are (Figure 14.1)[4], how confident they are about making a change and what their expectations are.
  - 'What are you hoping to get from coming to see me?'
  - 'On a scale of 1–10, how confident are you in being able to make this change? Why are you at that number and not zero?'
  - 'What benefit would you like to see from making this change?'

Information giving and PA prescription (if no medical clearance required)

- Reinforce *personalised* benefits, e.g. PA will help to lose weight, sleep better
- *If the patient is in the preparation phase*: Agree a prescription together (and ideally in written form) using the FITT framework (frequency, activity, time and type)
  - Moderate PA can be gauged using the 'talk test': '*You should be able to talk but not sing during the activity*'
  - This should be increased gradually

- **Safety net** with information about signs and symptoms which necessitate stopping PA and seeking medical help, including syncope, dizziness, severe shortness of breath (SOB), chest pain (CP), palpitations
- Recommend strategies to reduce sedentary time, e.g. get off the bus a stop early, take the stairs rather than the lift
- Personalise their immediate and long-term benefits of change
- Assist them by signposting to useful resources, e.g. websites, providing information leaflets and suggesting ways of tracking PA, e.g. pedometer or smart phone

Closing:

- Arrange a follow-up visit/phone call
- Provide contact details
- Make a referral to allied health professionals if appropriate, e.g. dietician, physiotherapist, smoking cessation services
- Check understanding
- Note: If the patient in precontemplation phase, it may not be appropriate to agree a PA prescription but to arrange a follow-up visit and provide written information

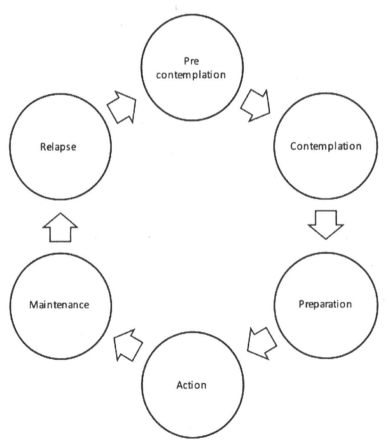

Figure 14.1 Stages of change model as defined by Prochaska and DiClemente [4].

Key points

- Use open-ended questions and motivational interviewing techniques, e.g. reflective listening, to establish the patient's readiness for change
- Personalise their activity prescription
- Ensure to risk assess and safety net for any medical contraindications

MEDICAL CLEARANCE

There are some occasions where individuals may require further investigation prior to initiating an exercise programme, or who may benefit from starting a supervised physical activity programme first. Historically, the exercise preparticipation health screening focussed on the number of cardiovascular disease risk factors and the presence of signs or symptoms of cardiovascular, metabolic and/or pulmonary disease. However, the American College of Sport and Exercise Medicine (ACSM) concluded in 2017 that this became a barrier to people who were otherwise safe to start light intensity physical activity (5). Whilst the previous guidelines only incorporated risk factors and signs or symptoms of disease, the updated guidelines (6) (Figure 14.2) incorporate an individual's:

a. Current physical activity level
b. History or signs or symptoms of cardiovascular, metabolic or renal disease
c. Desired intensity of physical activity

There are some validated questionnaires which can help inform a clinician during the process who may require further assessment, alongside a focussed history and examination, e.g. PAR-Q+. It also provides a validated and written documentation of risk assessment.

Regular physical activity is defined as 30 minutes of moderate-intensity activity on at least 3 days per week for at least 3 months.

Cardiovascular disease includes cardiac, peripheral vascular disease or cerebrovascular disease. Metabolic disease includes type 1 and 2 diabetes mellitus.

Major signs and symptoms suggestive of cardiovascular, metabolic and renal disease include:

- Pain in chest, neck, jaw
- Shortness of breath at rest or with mild exertion
- Dizziness or syncope
- Orthopnoea or paroxysmal nocturnal dyspnoea
- Ankle oedema
- Palpitations or tachycardia
- Intermittent claudication
- Heart murmur
- Unusual fatigue with activities of daily living (ADLs)

Although in the updated guidelines there is less emphasis on risk factors, their assessment should still be sought. Risk factors for CV disease include [7]:

- Age: Men ($\male$) ≥ 45 years; women ($\female$) ≥ 55 years
- Family history of myocardial infarction (MI) or sudden cardiac death (SCD) before

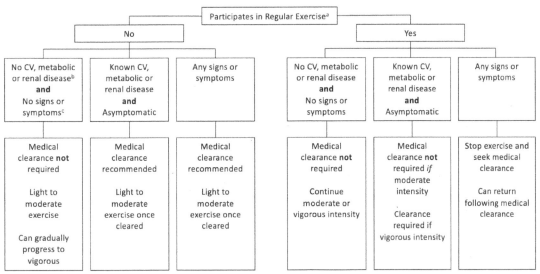

Figure 14.2 American College of Sports Medicine (ACSM) risk stratification flow diagram. See text for definition of (a) regular exercise and full criteria of (b) cardiovascular, metabolic or renal disease and (c) signs and symptoms of cardiovascular, metabolic and renal disease. (Abbreviation: CV = cardiovascular.) (Adapted from [6].)

55 years in ♂ first-degree relative or before 65 years ♀ first-degree relative
- Smoking: Current smoker or quit within the last 6 months
- BMI ≥ 30 kg/m^2 or waist circumference >102 cm for ♂ and >88 cm for ♀
- Hypertension ≥ 140 mmHg systolic or ≥90 mmHg diastolic or currently on anti-hypertensives
- Dyslipidaemia: Low density lipoproteins (LDL) ≥ 3.0 mmol/L, triglycerides ≥ 2.0 mmol/L or high density lipoproteins (HDL) < 1.0 mmol/L, total cholesterol ≥ 5.0 mmol/L or currently on lipid-lowering medication
- Impaired glucose tolerance: Fasting plasma glucose ≥ 6.1–6.9 mmol/L or ≥7.8–11 mmol/L 2 hours after 75 g oral glucose tolerance test (OGTT)

Patients with two or more risk factors are normally able to commence light to moderate-intensity physical activity but may require further investigation in some circumstances and before starting vigorous physical activity. The type of medical clearance is up to the discretion and clinical judgement of the physician but may include a resting or stress electrocardiogram (ECG), echocardiogram or other cardiac imaging including computed tomography (CT) or magnetic resonance imaging (MRI), nuclear medicine scans or angiography.

EXERCISE PRESCRIPTION WORKED EXAMPLES

DYSLIPIDAEMIA

"A 55-year-old male was recently found to have raised cholesterol on fasted bloods, results are shown in Table 14.2. He has a BMI of 28 and works as a lorry driver. He wants to take part in a 10-kilometre (km) sponsored charity walk at the end of the year. He currently walks about 3km three times a week and is asymptomatic for symptoms of major disease. He is on ramipril for high blood pressure. You are a General Practitioner (GP) and have a consultation to discuss physical activity and lifestyle with him."

Information gathering

- Establish the reason for attending or reason for referral and set the scene: *'I understand you would like to take part in a charity walk. Would it be OK if we discuss your physical activity today?'*
- Establish their current and previous physical activity – intensity, frequency and duration
  - Physical activity, exercise or sports participation?
  - Domestic chores, e.g. gardening, hoovering
  - Any occupational activity, e.g. unloading lorry
- Risk assessment:
  - Overweight on BMI and dyslipidaemia on bloods
  - Controlled hypertension
  - No current cardiovascular, respiratory or metabolic disease
  - No current symptoms of cardiovascular, respiratory or metabolic disease
  - As per ACSM guidelines, he does not require further clearance to participate in moderate-intensity activity such as walking
- Explore patient's **goals** (here to participate in charity walk), **preferred method** (e.g. group walking or individual) and any **barriers** (childcare, financial, time).
  - Use reflective listening: *'It sounds like you've already considered your goal of doing more walking this year'*

Table 14.2 Cardiometabolic blood results and reference ranges for patient		
Parameter	**Value**	**Reference range**
Cholesterol	6.0 mmol/L	<5.0 mmol/L
Triglycerides	1.8 mmol/L	0–1.7 mmol/L
HDL	1.2 mmol/L	1.2–3.0 mmol/L
LDL	3.1 mmol/L	1.0–3.0 mmol/L
HBA1c	35 mmol/mol	Non-diabetic <42 mmol/mol (below 6%) Diabetes ≥48 mmol/mol (6.5% or over)
Glucose	5.8 mmol/L	<7.0 mmol/L fasted <11.1 mmol/L 2 hours after OGTT
HDL, high dentisty lipoprotein; LDL, low density lipoprotein; OGTT, oral glucose tolerance test.		

- Calculate where in the 'Stages of Change' they are, how confident they are about making a change and what their expectations are.
  - 'On a scale of 1-10, how confident are you in being able to complete the charity walk? Why are you at that number and not zero?'
  - 'What benefit do you think you would have from doing it?'

Information giving and physical activity prescription

- Reinforce personal benefits, e.g. PA will help to control blood pressure, improve dyslipidaemia and potentially avoid having to start lipid-lowering drugs
- Agree a written prescription together using the FITT framework
  - Increase walk distance initially aiming to build up to 10 km by the end of the year. Progress slowly
  - Aim for moderate intensity, i.e. to be able to talk but not sing
  - Safety net with information about signs and symptoms which necessitate stopping PA, e.g. chest pain, palpitations, syncope
- Recommend strategies to reduce sedentary time, e.g. taking the stairs
- Signpost to useful resources, e.g. Walk4Life website, recommend a mobile phone app to monitor distance each week.

Closing:

- Arrange a follow-up visit/phone call
- Provide contact details
- Make a referral to a dietician given dyslipidaemia +/- liaise with GP regarding suitability for starting lipid lowering agents
- Check understanding and ask if he has any questions

PREGNANCY

"Heather is a 32-year-old woman who is 24 weeks pregnant with her first child. She has no underlying health conditions and is a non-smoker. She has experienced some morning sickness and fatigue in her first trimester and also has some pelvic girdle pain. Her BMI is 23. She has a history of depression but is not on any medication. She currently does an aerobics class once a week and has an office job. You are a specialist registrar in SEM and have a 10-minute slot to discuss PA during pregnancy with her."

Information gathering

- Establish their current and previous physical activity – both intensity, frequency and duration

Specific history:

- Any problems during pregnancy including cardiac and musculoskeletal such as pelvic girdle pain or obstetric abnormalities including placenta praevia or triplets
- Any diastasis recti
- Any previous complicated pregnancies or delivery

Risk assessment:

- Ask about contraindications including placenta praevia, premature rupture of membranes, cervical incompetence, persistent bleeding in second or third trimester, haemodynamically unstable cardiovascular disease, pre-eclampsia, intrauterine growth restriction (IUGR) (see Table 14.3) [8]
- Ask about symptoms during this pregnancy, including dizziness, marked fatigue, headaches
- Give PARmed-X for pregnancy
- Family history including SCD

Table 14.3 Absolute and relative contraindications for exercise during pregnancy

Absolute contraindications	Relative contraindications
• Haemodynamically significant heart disease	• Anaemia
• Restrictive lung disease	• Unevaluated maternal cardiac arrhythmia
• Incompetent cervix/cerclage	• Chronic bronchitis
• Multiple gestations at risk for premature labour	• Poorly controlled type 1 diabetes, hypertension, epilepsy or hyperthyroidism
• Persistent second or third trimester bleeding	• BMI >40 or <12 kg/m²
• Placenta praevia after 26 weeks	• Extreme sedentarism
• Current or previous history of premature labour	• Current intrauterine growth restriction
• Ruptured membranes	• Heavy smoker
• Pre-eclampsia	• Orthopaedic limitations
• Severe anaemia	

BMI, body mass index.

- Examination including height, weight, BMI, waist circumference, heart sounds, pulse, blood pressure (BP), urine dip, blood glucose (BM)
- Drug history, smoking and alcohol
- Find out the patient's **goals** (e.g. improve fatigue), **preferred method** (e.g. group or individual activity, indoor or outdoor) and any **barriers** (childcare, financial, time) – this will help you tailor the prescription.
- Calculate where in the 'Stages of Change' they are, how confident they are about making a change and what their expectations are.
  - *'What are you hoping to get from coming to see me?'*
  - *'On a scale of 1–10, how confident are you in being able to make this change'*
  - *'What benefit would you like to see from making this change?'*

Physical activity prescription

- Reinforce personalised benefits (e.g. reduces the risk of perinatal depression, improve pelvic girdle pain, lower gestational weight gain)
- Agree a prescription together (and ideally in written form) using the FITT framework (frequency, activity, time and type)
  - Useful to quote Chief Medical Officer guidelines of at least 150 minutes of moderate-intensity activity per week
  - Moderate PA can be gauged using the 'talk test': *'You should be able to talk but not sing during the activity'*
  - Non-weight bearing and low impact is normally best in pregnancy, e.g. swimming, but other exercises could include walking, running, yoga, dance
  - Avoid activities that exacerbate pelvic girdle pain
  - Women who are already active can continue what they are doing unless the activity is one of the specific precautions (see below)
- Highlight that moderate-intensity activity is safe in pregnancy but that there are some **pregnancy-specific precautions:** Do not perform exercises requiring Valsalva manoeuvre, avoid scuba diving, avoid supine position during the last 4 months of pregnancy, avoid excessive heat in first trimester, avoid activities that are high risk of impact to bump or danger of falling, incorporate pelvic floor exercises early
  - **Safety net** with information about signs and symptoms which necessitate stopping PA and seeking medical help – amniotic leak, vaginal bleeding, dizziness, painful uterine contractions, excessive SOB or CP

- Recommend strategies to reduce sedentary time, e.g. get off the bus a stop early, take the stairs rather than the lift
- Assist them by signposting to useful resources, e.g. Moving Medicine pregnancy resource, providing information leaflets and suggesting ways of tracking PA, e.g. pedometer or smartphone

Closing:

- Arrange a follow-up visit
- Provide contact details
- Make a referral to allied health professionals if appropriate, e.g. woman's physio for PGP
- Check understanding

SPECIAL GROUPS AND CONSIDERATIONS

Medications

ACE inhibitors – lower peripheral vascular resistance

Beta blockers – can reduce exercise capacity and heart rate responses, lower heart rate and cardiac output, greater risk of postural hypotension

Diuretics – risk of dehydration, postural hypotension, gout

Calcium channel blockers and nitrates – reduce cardiac output, can cause post-exercise hypotension. Recommend gradual cool down

NSAIDs – risk of renal impairment, UGI bleed, fluid retention

Insulin or sulphonylureas – risk of hypoglycaemia

Postpartum

- Identify any problems during pregnancy including cardiac and musculoskeletal such as pelvic girdle pain or obstetric abnormalities including placenta praevia or triplets
- Ask whether currently breastfeeding – breastfeed prior to exercise for comfort, ensure good hydration and wear a supportive bra
- Type of delivery and any complications
- Any diastasis recti

Hypertension

- Need full exercise screen and supervision if >200/115 mmHg
- Avoid Valsalva manoeuvre, e.g. isometric and upper body exercise, which raises blood pressure acutely
- Monitor at regular intervals to review ongoing need for antihypertensives
- Focus on lower resistance, higher reps

Peripheral vascular disease (PVD)

Patients with PVD have a high chance of having concomitant coronary artery disease, and further investigation, e.g. exercise stress testing may be appropriate prior to commencing an exercise programme.

- Aim for low impact, non-weight bearing activities
- Avoid exercise in cold air or water to reduce vasoconstriction
- Interval training with frequent rests is a good option – absence or reduction of pain will indicate when to increase duration or intensity (document ischaemic pain grades)
- Excellent foot care
- Ideally, in supervised rehabilitation programme

Diabetes mellitus

- High risk according to ACSM classification – require thorough medical exam and exercise test before moderate to vigorous physical activity
- Scrutinise insulin or medication regime to identify times to exercise with lowest risk of hypoglycaemia
- If proliferative retinopathy, avoid Valsalva or isometric weightlifting
- If peripheral neuropathy, avoid traumatic activities to feet

Osteoporosis

- Weight bearing or impact activities help to preserve bone mineral density (BMD). These include walking, jogging, dancing, stair climbing, aerobics, pilates, weights and balance exercises, e.g. tai chi
- Plyometrics should generally be avoided
- Non-weight bearing, e.g. swimming and cycling, do not preserve BMD as successfully
- Consider DEXA and metabolic bone specialist advice if low energy fracture after 40 years or significant risk factors

Older person

- Polypharmacy common – tailor exercise accordingly as above
- Resistance exercise and balance, particularly important to mitigate against sarcopenia and risk of falls – may necessitate physiotherapy referral
- If joint pain, non-weight bearing may be more appropriate initially

Cancer

- Avoid high impact and contact sport if presence of metastases as risk of pathological fracture
- If bone marrow transplant or low WCC, avoid communal areas
- No swimming if central line or having radiation
- If lymph node clearance, assess for lymphoedema. Low load weights and compression bandages may help
- Contraindications to exercising whilst having active treatment include: On the day of chemotherapy and within 24 hours, active infection, fever, diarrhoea and vomiting within 48 hours, new bony pain, haematological (Plt < 50, WCC < 3, Hb < 10)

REFERENCES

1. Bioethics, N.C.o., Public Health: Ethical Issues. 2007, Cambridge Publishers Ltd.
2. Craig, P., et al., Developing and evaluating complex interventions: the new Medical Research Council guidance. *BMJ.* 2008. 337: p. a1655.
3. Exercise Prescription in Health and Disease: a series of cases for medical students, The Faculty of Sport and Exercise Medicine (UK), Editor: United Kingdom.
4. Prochaska, J.O. and C.C. DiClemente, Stages and processes of self-change of smoking: toward an integrative model of change. *J Consult Clin Psychol.* 1983. 51(3): p. 390–5.
5. Whitfield, G.P., et al., Applying the ACSM Preparticipation Screening Algorithm to U.S. Adults: National Health and Nutrition Examination Survey 2001-2004. *Med Sci Sports Exerc.* 2017. 49(10): p. 2056–2063.
6. Riebe, D., et al., Updating ACSM's Recommendations for Exercise Preparticipation Health Screening, *Med Sci Sports Exerc.* 2015: United States. 47 (11) p. 2473–9.
7. Mozaffarian, D., et al., Heart disease and stroke statistics--2015 update: a report from the American Heart Association, *Circulation.* 2015; 131 (24): United States. 126(6): p. e29–322.
8. ACOG Committee Opinion No. 650: Physical Activity and Exercise During Pregnancy and the Postpartum Period, *Obstet Gynecol.* 2015: United States. p. e135–42.

15 Team and event medicine

INTRODUCTION

Scenarios specific to working in a professional sports setting have previously been assessed in Sport and Exercise Medicine (SEM) objective structured clinical examinations (OSCEs). This may include a discussion with a coach or event organiser to outline appropriate medical considerations for sporting events, tours or special circumstances such as altitude training. As with all the other stations, a clear structure is required, as well as knowledge or reference to the specific guidelines, clinical governance and organisations which dictate how you should manage and plan these particular events. Finally, specialist knowledge relevant to athletes, including pre-participation evaluation and doping, has also been assessed.

PITCH-SIDE MEDICINE

Stations have previously come up where you are given a trauma bag to rifle through and identify any pieces of kit that may be missing, followed by a discussion with a coach/organiser around medical planning for an event or match.

"You have been asked to cover as pitch-side doctor at a rugby match. Assess the current trauma bag and make a note of any additional kit you would like to include. Discuss with the coach your plans for an emergency action plan and organising medical services."

"You are providing medical cover at a one-day boxing tournament. Please list and explain the equipment you would like to bring and also what policies and protocols you would familiarise yourself with prior to the start."

Equipment

It is useful to remember a list of equipment in your head following the A, B, C, D, E approach.

Airway with cervical spine (C-spine) control:
- Portable suction and Magill forceps

- Airways including oropharyngeal (OP) and nasopharyngeal (NP)
- Supraglottic airways, e.g. i-gel®
- Emergency cricothyroid device
- Non-rebreathe mask
- Spinal collar

Breathing
- Bag valve mask
- Nebuliser

Circulation
- Cannulas
- Giving sets
- Crystalloid fluids, e.g. 0.9% NaCl
- Haemorrhage control pack
- Pelvic sling
- Intraosseous device

Disability
- Blood glucose monitor
- Pen torch
- Thermometer

Other
- Automated external defibrillator
- Musculoskeletal
  - Splints, crutches, Mediwrap®, strapping
- Wound care
  - Suture kit, gauze and dressings
- Stethoscope
- Longboard or split board with head blocks and straps (Figure 15.1)
- Active compression and cooling machine, e.g. Game Ready™

Medications (suggested but not limited to)
- Cardiac arrest medications: Adrenaline 1:10,000, amiodarone, atropine
- Adrenaline 1:100 for anaphylaxis/ Epipen®
- Oxygen cylinder
- Salbutamol
- Glucagon, concentrated glucose gel, 10% dextrose
- Hydrocortisone
- Chlorpheniramine
- Benzodiazepine, e.g. buccal midazolam
- Analgesia including Entonox or Penthrox

DOI: 10.1201/9781003163701-18

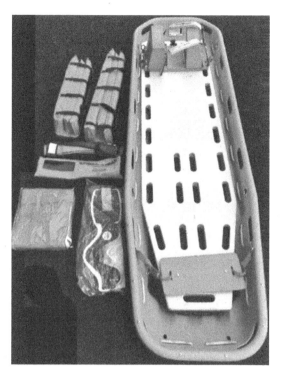

Figure 15.1 Pitch-side extrication equipment including (clockwise from *top left*) fracture splints, longboard and scoop with head blocks and straps, cervical collar, blanket and spider straps. (This figure was published in *A Comprehensive Guide to Sports Physiology and Injury Management*, Porter and Wilson, page 520, Copyright Elsevier, 2021.)

Additional medications outside of match days/emergency care may also include:
- Antibiotics including topical
- Intranasal steroids
- Antacids

Policies and protocols

1. Emergency action plan (for match and training days) (1)
   - Assigned roles for each individual, e.g. manual in-line stabilisation (MILS), airway, chest compressions
   - Dedicated time out prior to each match or training session to discuss roles
   - Practice moulages, e.g. extrication with cervical spine immobilisation
   - Identify entry and exit points including ambulance access
   - Identify the nearest trauma hospital and transit times
   - Outline debrief policy after every match or training
   - Discussion with paramedics and crowd doctor
   - Equipment and medication check

2. Communications
   - Printed contact details for personnel
   - Radio equipment and ensure working
   - Identify nearest unit and have printed materials of contacts for specialist ear, nose and throat (ENT), maxillofacial, plastics, paediatrics, orthopaedics, spinal and cardiac centres
   - Familiarise with referral pathways
   - Secure system for documentation
   - Preparation of SAMPLE forms for each player and member of staff ready for handover

3. Other
   - Anti-doping – familiarise with procedures and assigned room and personnel
   - Infection control
   - Sharps injuries protocol

TEAM TRAVEL

"You are the team doctor for the national hockey team who are due to play in the world championships in Oman in 6 months' time. You have a meeting with the head coach to discuss planning for the trip. Please explain what things need to be organised from a medical point of view prior to and during the trip. You have 10 minutes to prepare, and then 10 minutes for discussion."

The best way to approach this station is by having some structure to your answer. One way is to divide your answer into tasks *before* travel, tasks *during* travel and tasks *after* travel. Remember to consider staff as well as players in your plan and tailor the strategy according to the country you are to visit (i.e. climate considerations, vaccinations, hygiene, etc.) and the team you are travelling with (para-athletes, adolescents). It is helpful to have an acronym as an *aide memoire* so that you can plan your answer under pressure without missing out key aspects. You can devise your own one or use the one suggested below.

Before travel

Information gathering: How many athletes, how many staff, how long is the trip, what time of year, funding, etc.

Acronym: TEAMPRO

T	Travel destination
E	Equipment
A	Administration
M	Medicines
P	Pre-competition camp
R	Repatriation Planning
O	Other

Travel destination

- Season and altitude – if very hot or humid to consider sunscreen requirements and additional fluid and electrolyte replacement, factor in acclimatisation
- Are any diseases endemic? Use website **TravelHealthPro/National Travel Health Network and Centre (NaTHNaC)** (or your home country equivalent) which will advise on what vaccinations are required or recommended and if malaria prophylaxis required
  - Oman is high risk for food and waterborne infectious diseases, such as cholera, hepatitis A, travellers' diarrhoea or typhoid. Consider prophylactic antibiotics for staff. Consider alcohol gel for each player and educate team on scrupulous handwashing
- Water supplies – Can you drink the tap water? Bottled water recommended in Oman
- Security – crime levels, terrorism threat, organise airport transfers
- Jet lag – planning of travel with consideration of changing time zones. Ideally, players should have enough time to acclimatise to the environment as well as time difference

Equipment

- Find out the airline rules on weight allowance
- Medical equipment baggage waiver and ensure all items listed and available for inspection, e.g. defibrillator
- Organise whether you will need to carry gases with you and appropriate paperwork

Administration

- Insurance and indemnity – repatriation plan with insurance
- Parental permission if under 18 and safeguarding processes in place
- Pre-prepare SAMPLE forms for each player and staff member
- Construct emergency action plans for each venue
- Ensure all therapeutic use exemptions (TUEs) in place
- Documentation for medication and pressurised gases

Medicines

- Ensure prescription for any prescribed medications and sufficient supplies.
- Controlled drugs may need an application for licence via the **Home Office (Drug and Firearm Licensing Unit)** (www.gov.uk) or your home country equivalent. Need to fill out an application form with a letter proving prescription for player *at least 10 days prior to travel. This is required if travelling for 3 months or more.*
- Visiting country's restrictions on medications, e.g. opiates
- Ensure TUEs in place

Pre-competition camp (at least 6 weeks prior)

- An opportunity to educate players and staff on country-specific information – water supplies, vaccinations, climate, anti-doping guidelines
- Perform pre-travel medical assessment and prepare SAMPLE forms
- Obtain information on all recent injuries/illnesses and obtain next of kin details
- Ensure all TUEs in place

Repatriation planning and secondary care facilities

- Ideally, make an advanced visit to competition location to establish the location of hospitals and major trauma centres
- Find out transfer times to secondary care and establish process for emergency repatriation with a travel insurance company and plan for staff division should this occur
- Evacuation plan

Other: Anything else

During travel

- Medical bag, weight allowance, bring medications for travel sickness and analgesia
- Food and water for the duration of journey, advise against alcohol or caffeine
- Thrombo-embolus deterrent (TED) stockings and encourage the regular movement of lower limbs to prevent a deep vein thrombosis (DVT)
- Ear plugs and eye masks for sleep
- Jet lag – advise to set watch to destination time as soon as possible

At destination

- Establish medical room and establish appointment sheet and hours
- Provide contact number to players and have back up in case you become unwell
- Establish sources for ice
- At each venue, establish roles with hosting staff and practice moulage at venues
- Assess daily stock of medication and equipment

On return

- Medical debriefing
- Assessment of quantities of medications and equipment used
- Remind staff and players for symptoms on return of DVT or diarrhoeal illness

EVENT MEDICINE

"You have been appointed Chief Medical Officer (CMO) for a National Youth Games tournament involving rugby, football and hockey. Please go through considerations and planning to the event manager."

"You are in charge of planning a trail running event in the Lake District. There will be 5,000 runners. Outline the planning considerations in your role as CMO."

Similar to the above, the best way to approach this station is by having some structure to your answer. An acronym commonly used in the military is TEPID-OIL (Training, Equipment, Personnel, Information, Doctrine and Concepts, Organisation, Infrastructure and Logistics). Another suggestion is PREPARE (Provision, Equipment, Personnel, Administration, Read [Pre-Event Information], Environment).

Information gathering

You may wish to clarify with the event manager the number of athletes and spectators and key infrastructure information such as indoor facilities.

Outline plan using TEPID-OIL

Training

- Staff education on event, demographic of competitors, number of competitors and spectators
- Epidemiology of injuries and illnesses previously
- Staff training in emergency action plan
- Staff training on communications and documentation

Equipment + environment

- Medical tent, beds and stations
- ABC + defibrillator
- Ambulance + paramedic if >5,000 people – in the UK, see the 'Green Guide' (2) or International Federation Guide (3) for numbers
  - E.g. One ambulance for >5,000 people, one ambulance, paramedic and ambulance officer if 5–25,000 people, if >25,000 people then also need major incident equipment vehicle
  - At least two first aiders, one first aider/ 1,000 people up to 20,000

- Point of care sodium testing (e.g. i-STAT®),
- Personal protective equipment (PPE), sharps bins
- Medications all in date
- Communication systems – radios, computers
- Musculoskeletal equipment, e.g. brace, tape, splints
- Protocol for handling and disposing of human products

Personnel

- Staff – doctors, physiotherapists, paramedics, nurses, stewards, CMO ideally should be MIMMS (Major Incident Medical Management and Support) trained
- Crowd doctor trained in immediate care if >2,000 spectators
- Ensure doctors have appropriate pitch-side care certificate and sufficient experience
- Curriculum Vitae and indemnity for staff
- Green guide/mandatory requirements of international federation
- Define roles and training beforehand
- Arrange training sessions including key diagnoses and arrival and departure time
- Passes for access to medical tent

Infrastructure

- Nearest trauma unit, neurosurgical, transfer times, helicopter support
- Entry and exit routes
- Contact numbers

Doctrine and concepts

- Standard operating procedures (SOPs) and protocols – send out ahead of time
- Hypothermia management
- Hyponatraemia management
- Cardiopulmonary resuscitation (CPR)

Organisation

- Insurance
- Indemnity
- Contracts with clear roles
- Major incident plan
- Pre-event meeting with staff

Information

- Send out to athletes ahead of time advising on nutrition, clothes, travel
- Training for staff pre-race–SOPs

Logistics

- Weather, altitude, cancellation policy
- Day, date and time – ensure no clashes with other events

- Access and exit routes for people and ambulances
- Local hospital and transport times

Other: Administration

- Agreement with organising body
- Insurance
- Medical log in system and training
- Injury forms
- Daily venue reports
- CMO role – contract
- Adverse Event protocol for catastrophic injuries that addresses confidentiality and medical reporting

PRE-PARTICIPATION EVALUATION (PPE)

"You are the doctor for a Championship Football Team. You have been asked to conduct a pre-participation evaluation on a new player. You have not received any previous information about their past medical history or injuries yet."

History:

- Demographic – age, position, competition level, dominant leg, how many matches in the last 12 months
- Past medical history
  - General – infections, concussion
  - Cardiovascular – specifically ask about chest pain, shortness of breath (SOB), palpitations, syncope, dizziness, blackouts, ankle swelling, orthopnea
  - Respiratory – SOB, wheeze, cough, fatigue
  - Musculoskeletal/injury – any injury requiring >4 weeks out, surgery, injections, ask about each joint specifically
  - Psychiatric – mood disorder, alcohol, eating disorder
- Family history
  - Sudden cardiac death (SCD; also ask about unexplained deaths, drowning, syncope in family)
  - Coronary heart disease (CHD; first-degree relative male < 55 years, female < 65 years)
  - Other: Cardiomyopathy, hypertension, Marfan's syndrome, diabetes mellitus (DM)
- Drug history – including supplements, over the counter (OTC) medications, recreational, alcohol and allergies

Examination:

- Height, weight and body mass index (BMI), body fat %

- Observations: Heart rate (HR) and blood pressure (BP)
- Cardiovascular – heart sounds, murmurs, jugular venous pressure (JVP), central and peripheral pulses including femoral delay and bruits
- Respiratory – percuss and auscultate
- Abdominal examination
- Check for features of Marfan's syndrome
- Musculoskeletal assessment including range of movement (ROM) using goniometer, strength, isokinetic dynamometer
  - Spine and pelvis
  - Hip – ROM and pain
  - Muscles – adductors, hamstrings, iliopsoas, rectus femoris, iliotibial band
  - Knee – ROM, Lachman's test, collaterals, menisci
  - Foot and ankle – ROM, Achilles tendon, anterior drawer
- Functional assessment, e.g. single leg hop distance, jump height

Investigations:

- 12-lead electrocardiogram (ECG) and echocardiogram (4) – cardiologist to interpret
  - Left ventricular hypertrophy, QTC interval
  - Left ventricular function
  - Cardiomyopathy, Wolf Parkinson White

Note: Despite being advocated by the International Olympic Committee (5), the level of athlete cardiac screening differs worldwide due to variable acceptance of its efficacy, reliability and cost (6). In the UK, mandatory cardiac screening is carried out across a range of professional sports including but not limited to Team Great Britain (GB) Olympic and Paralympic athletes, England Rugby Football Union, Lawn Tennis Association, Premiership and Championship football clubs and the English Cricket Board, e.g. by the institution screening via cardiac risk in the young (CRY) – note may have implications on life insurance and mortgage.

- Other: Eye check with optician, dental check, skin assessment
- Mental health questionnaire screening
- Bloods: Full blood count (FBC), urea and electrolytes (U&E), liver function tests (LFTs), thyroid function tests (TFTs), bone profile, vitamin D, iron studies

Final summary

- Eligible to play
- Eligible but follow up needed
- Play not recommended
- Advise not to play awaiting ECG and echo results

EXPEDITION MEDICINE AND ALTITUDE

"You have been asked to help arrange a high-altitude training camp abroad for elite distance runners at an altitude of approximately 3000-2500 metres. You have a meeting with the head coach who wants to discuss the planning of the trip and the possible specific medical problems they could encounter at altitude."

Information gathering

- Find out how many athletes, level of competition, aims of training, staff attending, any athletes with the previous history of altitude sickness?
- Information of destination, e.g. average temperature (risk of hypothermia), endemic illnesses

Information giving

- Acclimatisation advice (7)
  - Need minimum 2 weeks acclimatisation if >2,500 m (8,000 feet), then add a week for every additional 600 m
  - This may involve flying in at altitude and spending 2-3 days at that altitude before ascending
  - Avoid rapid ascent >500 m/day
  - Above 3,000 m, no more than >300 m increase in sleeping altitude per day with a rest day every 3rd day, in which aim to sleep at the same elevation for at least one additional night
  - Risk assessment required (see Table 15.1)
- General recommendations
  - Avoid alcohol and opiates

- Maintain hydration and nutrition rich in protein and carbohydrate
- Training considerations
  - Live high, train low (so that exercise intensity can be reached for adaptation)
  - Note: Some are non-responders
  - Monitor training - rate of perceived exertion (RPE), iron status
  - Improvement in oxygen carrying capacity lasts approximately 3 weeks so it is important to factor this in with anticipated date of competition
- Medical conditions at altitude
  - Altitude sickness - above 2,500 m
    - Symptoms: Headache, insomnia, anorexia, nausea, SOB, morning or nocturnal symptoms, e.g. Cheyne-Stokes breathing
    - Can use Lake Louise score (8) to assess, which incorporates headache, gastrointestinal symptoms, fatigue or weakness, dizziness and difficulty sleeping
    - Consider acetazolamide 125 mg BD as prophylaxis (private prescription) in those with previous altitude sickness - start 2 days before ascent and stop below 2,500 m
      1. Side effects: Altered taste, paraesthesia, polyuria
      2. Diuresis and excrete sodium bicarbonate causing metabolic acidosis and hyperventilation
      3. Contraindicated in glaucoma, hypokalaemia, hyponatraemia, renal or hepatic impairment, pregnancy or allergy to sulphonamides. Can also interact with high dose

Table 15.1 Risk categories for acute mountain sickness as per the Wilderness Medicine Society (7)	
Risk	**Details**
Low	• Individuals with no prior history of altitude illness and ascending to ≤2,800 m • Individuals taking ≥2 days to arrive at 2,500–3,000 m with subsequent increases in sleeping elevation <500 m per day and an extra day for acclimatisation every 1,000 m
Moderate	• Individuals with a history of AMS ascending to 2,500–2,800 m in one day • Individuals with no history of AMS ascending to >2,800 m in one day • All individuals ascending >500 m/day (in sleeping elevation) at altitudes above 3,000 m but with an extra day for acclimatisation every 1,000 m
High	• Individuals with a history of AMS ascending to >2,800 m in one day • All individuals with a history of HACE or HAPE • All individuals ascending to >3,500 m in one day • All individuals ascending >500 m/day (in sleeping elevation) above 3,000 m without extra days for acclimatisation • Very rapid ascents (e.g. <7-day ascents of Mt. Kilimanjaro)

AMS, acute mountain sickness; HACE, high altitude cerebral oedema; HAPE, high altitude pulmonary oedema.

aspirin, cardiac glycosides, antihypertensives and lithium
- High altitude pulmonary oedema (HAPE)
  - SOB, cough, frothy pink sputum
  - Management: Descend, nifedipine, oxygen
- High altitude cerebral oedema
  - Confusion, headache, ataxia, reduced consciousness/ Glasgow Coma Scale (GCS)
  - Management: Descend, oxygen, dexamethasone
- Extrication planning and communications should this occur
  - Also, frostbite/frostnip/hypothermia
- Equipment required, e.g. Acetazolamide? Oxygen, vaccinations, etc.
- Contraindications to altitude: Pregnancy, polycythaemia, sickle cell disease, previous altitude-related illness, relative energy deficiency in sport (RED-S), refractory eye surgery. Also ask about high BP, heart, kidney or lung problems, DM, anaemia, glaucoma, obstructive sleep apnoea (OSA) which can worsen at altitude
- NHS choices and NaTHNaC give good advice on altitude illness
- Ensure travel insurance adequately covers itinerary and activities with full disclosure of planned elevation

Closing

- Summarise what you have said
- Arrange follow up for risk assessment of athletes
- Detail administration to complete, including insurance, medications, equipment, e.g. oxygen

DIVING MEDICINE

"You are the doctor for a marine diving conservation project in Mexico. A colleague comes to alert you to a diver who recently surfaced from a deep dive who is complaining of shortness of breath and joint pains. Please assess."

Decompression illness (DCI), or generalised barotrauma, is caused when inert nitrogen gas dissolved in tissue under pressure precipitates out of solution and forms bubbles within the venous, lymphatic system or body tissues rather than being eliminated by the lungs. It typically presents within 6 hours of surfacing but can present up to 48 hours after diving.

Arterial gas embolism occurs when nitrogen bubbles enter the arterial circulation, either via a patent foramen ovale or directly with pulmonary barotrauma.

Clinical features of decompression illness:

- General – malaise, headache, lethargy

- Musculoskeletal – joint pain: 'the bends' – initially in large joints
- Dermatological – mottled rash (cutis marmorata), pruritus
- Cardiopulmonary – chest pain (pleuritic or retrosternal), SOB, cough, haemoptysis
- Neurological
  - Audiovestibular (labyrinth damage with vertigo, deafness, tinnitus and nystagmus)
  - Sensory disturbance such as paraesthesia and tingling, motor abnormalities including hemiplegia
  - Amnesia, confusion, vision abnormalities, personality change, seizures

Clinical features of pulmonary barotrauma:

- Cardiopulmonary – chest pain and dyspnoea secondary to surgical emphysema, pneumothorax or pneumomediastinum
- Neurological – sudden onset after surfacing, e.g. confusion, seizures, coma secondary to reduced cerebral circulation

History:

- Current symptoms and any improvement with oxygen
- Timing and onset of symptoms
- What type of circuit was used (open circuit most common)
- Details of dive – depth, duration, safety stops, any rapid ascents (air embolism)
- Recent dive history: Multiple dives, how many consecutive days diving
- Other: recent flights, alcohol use, previous DCI

Examination:

After initial ABCDE assessment, examination should also include a thorough clinical examination with a focus on the cardiopulmonary, neurological, musculoskeletal and dermatological assessment.

Management of decompression illness:

- ABCDE assessment with high flow oxygen via non-rebreathe mask
- Manage patient supine or in left lateral position
- Establish intravenous (IV) access and take bloods for FBC, U&E, LFTs, glucose, troponin and creatine kinase (CK)
- Give 0.9% NaCl
- Perform ECG and chest X-ray (CXR) if available
- Seizures may require benzodiazepine infusion
- Avoid opiates or glucose containing fluids
- Call your national diving accident helpline or helpline of the country you are in
- Urgently refer to the nearest hyperbaric medicine unit. Long-distance repatriation requires air transport presence

DOPING

"An international-level rugby player comes to see you as team doctor whilst on tour in South Africa and discloses that he has been using testosterone. The opening match is in 2 days and he is second batsman. He asks you not to disclose to the coach. Please discuss your plan with the player."

"On pre-season medical a player states that he has been taking a creatine supplement for the last 2 months, on advice from another player. Please have a conversation with the player regarding the supplement and provide wider doping counselling."

1. **Information gathering**
   - Open conversation and set the scene
   - Explore their reason for taking, e.g. performance enhancement, inadvertent, recovery
   - Take a history: Duration, frequency, dose, method, side effects, reason, are they distributing/dealing to others? When did they last take?
     - Time for cocaine to leave system: 3–5 days
     - Time for testosterone to leave the system: up to 45 days
   - Have they got wider psychiatric issues, e.g. depression, body dysmorphia, addiction
2. **Examination**
   - Health of player paramount
   - Offer to do the examination and basic observations
   - May have to perform investigations, e.g. bloods, liver screen depending on substance used. However, caution as this could be interpreted as aiding and abetting
3. **Educate patient**
   - Each athlete has a **strict liability** for any substances found in their body, whether intentional or unintentional (inadvertent doping) (9)
   - Commonest cause of inadvertent doping is contaminated supplements
     - Use *Informed Sport* (https://sport. wetestyoutrust.com) to check supplements and advise the athlete to carry paper with brand, batch number and ingredients with them
     - Use *Global DRO* (www.globaldro. com) to check medication (apllies to UK, United States, Canada, Australia, Japan)
   - Explain that they are risking their career, health, and disqualification of the team, by knowingly doping. Explain safe and legal alternatives to enhance performance/improve recovery, etc.

Ethical issues

- Some players may ask you to monitor their bloods to ensure no further harm whilst they continue to take the prohibited substances or prescribe diuretic to cover up – this is aiding and abetting, which is prohibited
- If they ask you not to disclose to anyone, e.g. coach, as per Good Medical Council (GMC) guidance, you should not break confidentiality. There are a few circumstances where you can do so:
  - Unless by not doing so poses a risk to athlete or others
  - Safeguarding concern
  - If an athlete admits to taking illegal drugs, to justify disclosure, the seriousness of a crime would need to represent a real risk to public safety
- You may have to advise the coach that the player is not available for selection due to a medical reason but unable to specifically disclose the reason due to confidentiality
- Sensible measures would be to check your own and players contract if there is a clause stating the player has to disclose medical reasons for non-selection to coach. Also discussing with medical defence union or senior colleague in confidence for advice going forward

Closing

- Agree plan with player going forward, e.g. in case of testosterone not available for selection currently, but you do not have to disclose reason
- Make a plan for addressing reasons for using in the first place
- Arrange follow-up plans and signpost to resources, e.g. World Anti-Doping Agency (WADA), UK Anti-Doping (UKAD) and 100% Me app
- There is a wider education issue here as other team members may also be using – arrange educational session and meeting with specific players if necessary

"A player recently selected to represent Team GB in athletics has become part of the national testing pool. They take a salbutamol inhaler. There have recently been some doping violations in the team secondary to inadvertent doping with unregulated supplements. You have been asked to give them some information about doping as part of their induction."

Information gathering

- What do they already know about prohibited substances and the WADA guidelines?

- How long have they been taking a salbutamol inhaler, what dose and what indication?
- Any other prescribed medications, OTC medications or supplements?

Information giving

- Therapeutic Use Exemption (TUE) criteria:
  - Significant health problems without taking prohibited substance or method
  - No performance enhancement
  - No reasonable alternative
- Inhaled salbutamol is allowed (maximum 1,600 micrograms over 24 hours in divided doses not to exceed 800 micrograms over 12 hours starting from any dose). The presence in urine of salbutamol in excess of 1,000 ng/mL is not consistent with therapeutic use of the substance
- International-level athletes must apply to the International Federation and National Level athletes apply to their home country national anti-doping organisation equivalent (national level athletes in the UK apply to UKAD) complete with all medical information, tests, laboratory results, imaging and clinical information
  - Use the Anti-Doping Administration and Management System (ADAMS), which is a centralised platform managed by WADA. This will also be used to record their whereabouts
  - This should be prospective apart from if emergency treatment is required
  - There are in competition versus out of competition banned substances
- Violations include (10)
  - Deliberate cheating using banned substances or methods, e.g. no more than 100 mL of intravenous fluids and/or injections over 12 hours (unless as part of hospital treatment)
  - Evading testing
  - Inadvertent doping
  - Complicity – if involved in a violation committed by another person
  - Prohibited association – liaising or associating with individual guilty of a doping violation
  - Cumulative whereabouts violations – 3 missed tests or filing failures in 12 months
- Reasons an athlete may reasonably delay testing: Participate in awards ceremony, media commitment, compete in further competition, warm down, training session, obtain medical treatment, locate representative, obtain photo identification

- Inadvertent doping is a common cause for violations. If an athlete has used contaminated products by mistake, they would need to provide substantial proof to avoid a penalty. To check for specific substances:
  a. Use *Informed Sport* (https://sport.wetestyoutrust.com) to check supplements and advise the athlete to carry paper with brand, batch number and ingredients with them
  b. Use *Global DRO* (www.globaldro.com) to check medication (applies to the UK, United States, Canada, Australia, Japan)
- Outline testing procedure, i.e. Bottle A and B and filling in associated paperwork.

Closing

- Ask if the athlete has any questions
- Arrange follow-up plans and signpost to resources, e.g. UKAD, WADA
- Engage with education, e.g. 100% me app
- Arrange follow-up and plan to organise a TUE for their salbutamol

REFERENCES

1. Shah R, Wilson CAJ. Creating a model of best practice: The match day emergency action protocol. *Br J. Sports Med.* 2018;52(23): 1535–36.
2. *The Guide to Safety at Sports Grounds (The Green Guide)*, Department for Culture, Media and Sport, Football Licensing Authority, 6th edition, 2018.
3. *Health Care Guidelines for International Federation Events*, Association of Summer Olympic International Federations (ASOIF's) Medical and Scientific Consultative Group (AMSCG), 2020.
4. Dvorak J, et al. Development and implementation of a standardized precompetition medical assessment of international elite football players–2006 FIFA World Cup Germany. *Clin J Sport Med.* 2009;19(4):316–21.
5. Ljungqvist A, et al. The International Olympic Committee (IOC) consensus statement on periodic health evaluation of elite athletes, *Clin J Sport Med.* 2009;19(5):347–65.
6. Dhutia H, MacLachlan H. Cardiac screening of young athletes: A practical approach to sudden cardiac death prevention. *Curr Treat Options Cardiovasc Med.* 2018;20(10):85.
7. Luks AM, et al. Wilderness Medical Society Clinical Practice Guidelines for the prevention and treatment of acute altitude illness: 2019 update. *Wilderness Environ Med.* 2019;30(4S):S3–18.
8. Roach RC, et al. The 2018 Lake Louise acute mountain sickness score. *High Alt Med Biol.* 2018;19(1):4–6.
9. *The 2021 UK Anti-Doping Rules*, UK Anti-Doping Authority (UKAD), Editor, 2021.
10. *World Anti-Doping Code*, World Anti-Doping Agency (WADA), 2021.

PART C

Emergencies

16 Medical emergencies

INTRODUCTION

Assessment and management of an acutely unwell patient is a key skill required as a sport and exercise medicine physician. Inevitably in the specialty, you are more likely to have to deal with these scenarios in a pre-hospital or pitch-side setting. Previous objective structured clinical examination (OSCE) stations have therefore commonly reflected this and as well as a slick and comprehensive assessment, management will often include appropriate secondary care referral and 'packaging', i.e. making a patient suitable for transfer and handover. To become proficient in these types of stations both for an examination and real-life, simulation is the best form of practice. Sitting an approved emergency care course in sport a few months before taking the exam will prime and prepare you with the foundations of assessment and management and give you an example of the sort of conditions that may arise. These include but are not limited to Pre-Hospital Immediate Care in Sport (PHICIS), Advanced Trauma Medical Management in Football (ATMMiF) and Immediate Medical Management of the Field of Play (IMMFP) of which there is cross recognition of their qualification. Finally, practising relevant scenarios with peers is also an excellent way to prepare for these type of stations. With sufficient preparation, by the time of the exam, you should feel confident in being able to perform an A to E assessment in your sleep and deal with the major diagnoses detailed in this chapter.

ASSESSMENT OF THE ACUTELY UNWELL PATIENT

PITCH-SIDE ASSESSMENT

In practice, the pitch-side assessment is not the same as one we do in a hospital setting due to the nature of the environment, e.g. difficulty in auscultating chest above the noise of a stadium crowd and the impracticality in performing certain specialist investigations. The purpose of the pitch-side assessment is to assess any life or limb-threatening injuries. Your assessment should include the standard ABCDE approach with consideration of the cervical spine (C-spine) and be sufficient for you to assess the patient safely and deal with major complications before transfer to a quieter setting such as the medical room to perform a more detailed assessment. Remember in your ABCDE approach not to move onto the next section of your assessment until you have addressed any problems with the one before, e.g. you should not move on to assess breathing if the patient does not have a secure airway.

"You are the doctor for a rugby team and a player goes down in the scrum. It is not clear from bystanders or the video replay of the mechanism. You run on to assess him. He is breathing with a pulse but not responding to you. You have a physiotherapist and three other members of staff available to help if needed"

1. Is it safe to approach?
2. Apply manual in-line stabilisation (MILS) unless mechanism of injury (MOI) clearly suggests improbable cervical spine injury
3. Call for help and ask them to take MILS whilst you conduct further assessment
4. ABCDE assessment:

Airway:

- Check for signs of obstruction and ascertain patency, e.g. listen for stridor or snoring
- Open mouth. Suction under direct supervision if liquid or use Magill forceps if solid obstruction, e.g. tooth
- If airway compromised, perform jaw thrust (head tilt chin lift contraindicated if suspected C-spine injury)

DOI: 10.1201/9781003163701-20

- Consider correctly sized adjuncts such as nasopharyngeal airway or oropharyngeal airway (see the box titled 'Sizing adjuncts')
- Escalate to supraglottic air way +/– surgical if required
- Apply high flow oxygen (15 L via a non-rebreathe mask)

Sizing adjuncts

Nasopharangeal (NP): Size of right nostril. Insert with bevel of the tip towards nasal septum

Oropharangeal (OP): Angle of mandible to mid-point of incisors – insert the correct way round with tongue depressor

Breathing:

- Assess respiratory rate (RR)
- Assess expansion – is it equal and of normal volume?
- Assess for pain on palpation of thorax

Circulation:

- Feel for radial pulse
  - If no radial pulse, feel for a carotid pulse → if not present start cardiopulmonary resuscitation (CPR)
  - If no radial pulse but carotid pulse is present, cannulate with large bore cannula, e.g. 16 g (grey) into a large vein such as antecubital fossa and give 250 mL bolus of crystalloid, e.g. 0.9% NaCl, and reassess

Disability: Assess using AVPU (**A**lert? Responds to **V**oice? Responds to **P**ain? **U**nresponsive?)

Exposure:

- Top to toe assessment including palpating for major trauma and/or haemorrhage 'on the floor and 5 more'
  - Thorax (assessed in Breathing)
  - Abdomen
  - Retroperitoneal
  - Pelvis
  - Four long bones of the limbs

Once any intervention has been performed or any change in status of the patient, then start from the beginning and reassess again.

Call for an ambulance early, e.g. if they will require investigations in hospital or secondary care input.

Extrication:

Once ABCDE has been performed, the patient can be extricated to medical room or ambulance:

- Suitable kit to extricate, e.g. longboard or split
- Triple immobilise with C spine collar (correctly sized from infra mental line to top of trapezius), blocks and straps. Reassess the airway after applying the collar
- It requires five people to safely get a patient onto a longboard or split, with person on MILS giving commands, three to turn their body and one to place the board underneath
  - E.g. For the split board the team can rotate on command to 15°, and then lower together once the board placed underneath
- Tighten body straps prior to head blocks and head straps

MEDICAL ROOM ASSESSMENT

"Once moved to the medical room the player is breathing but appears confused."

Perform ABCDE assessment again

Airway: Recheck as above

Breathing:

- RR
- Pain on palpation
- Expansion

Also:

- Percussion
- Auscultation

Circulation:

- Radial pulse – rate and character
- Blood pressure, if available
- Capillary refill (should be <2 seconds)

Disability:

- Glasgow Coma Scale (GCS; using a chart is easier than from memory – see the box titled 'Glasgow Coma Scale') with pupillary assessment
- Perform a bedside blood sugar (BM)

Exposure:

- Top to toe assessment as above
- Temperature if available

Glasgow Coma Scale

Eyes (4)

- Spontaneous 4
- To sound 3
- To pressure 2
- None 1

Verbal (5)

- Orientated 5
- Confused 4
- Words 3
- Sounds 2
- None 1

Motor (6)

- Obey commands 6
- Localising 5
- Normal flexion 4
- Abnormal flexion 3
- Extension 2
- None 1

Secondary survey

History (use SAMPLE mnemonic):

- S – Signs/symptoms
- A – Allergies
- M – Medications
- P – Past medical history
- L – Last oral intake
- E – Events leading up to illness/injury

Full physical examination:

- Re-evaluation
- Document observations

Transfer to definitive care:

- Ensure safe to move
- Handover
- Good documentation
- Contact with receiving hospital

Handover to ambulance using ATMIST:

- A – age of patient
- T – timing of injury
- M – mechanism of injury
- I – injuries sustained or suspected
- S – signs including observations
- T – treatment given

"This is a 28-year-old rugby player who approximately an hour ago sustained a blow to the head and went down in the scrum. We are unable to clear his C-spine at present due to confusion. A–E assessment reveals no life or limb threatening injuries. His vital observations are stable and to date he is being given high-flow oxygen 15L via non-rebreathe mask and has a cervical spine collar in situ."

MEDICAL EMERGENCIES

ANAPHYLAXIS

"A member of staff alerts you to a 21-year-old hockey player who has some difficulty breathing after eating an energy bar in the sports ground cafeteria. Their lips appear swollen. Please assess."

A rapid, immunological, multisystem reaction that can occur after drug ingestion (e.g. penicillin, angiotensin converting enzyme inhibitors [ACEi]), a wasp sting or certain foods, e.g. nuts.

Clinical features:

- Respiratory: shortness of breath (SOB), hoarseness, stridor, cough, cyanosis, oedema
- Cardiovascular: Hypotension, tachycardia, syncope, clammy
- Gastrointestinal: Abdominal pain, diarrhoea and vomiting
- Cutaneous: Urticaria, angioedema, pruritis

Management (Figure 16.1):

- ABCDE approach and call an ambulance
- High flow oxygen 15 L/min via a non-rebreathe mask and lie patient flat/elevate the legs
- If angioedema or wheeze:
  - Adrenaline (1:1000) 500 micrograms intra-muscular (IM) (can repeat after 5 minutes)
  - Hydrocortisone 200 mg IM or intravenous (IV)
  - Chlorphenamine 10 mg IM or IV (second-line measure used after achieving cardio-respiratory stability)
- Hypotension
  - Cannulate and give bolus of 500 mL 0.9% NaCl
  - Stop IV colloid

Monitor (if available): Pulse oximetry, electrocardiogram (ECG) and blood pressure (BP).

Re-review using ABCDE approach after each intervention given.

There is a high risk of airway compromise and patients may require early intubation. All patients require hospital admission and monitoring for at least 8 hours as a biphasic response can occur.

Follow up:

- Inform General Practitioner (GP)
- Any significant attacks should have mast cell tryptase measured in hospital and require allergy clinic referral on discharge

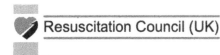

Resuscitation Council (UK)

Anaphylaxis algorithm

Anaphylactic reaction?

↓

Airway, Breathing, Circulation, Disability, Exposure

↓

Diagnosis - look for:
- Acute onset of illness
- Life-threatening Airway and/or Breathing and/or Circulation problems [1]
- And usually skin changes

↓

- **Call for help**
- Lie patient flat
- Raise patient's legs

↓

Adrenaline [2]

↓

When skills and equipment available:
- Establish airway
- High flow oxygen
- IV fluid challenge [3]
- Chlorphenamine [4]
- Hydrocortisone [5]

Monitor:
- Pulse oximetry
- ECG
- Blood pressure

---

[1] **Life-threatening problems:**
Airway: swelling, hoarseness, stridor
Breathing: rapid breathing, wheeze, fatigue, cyanosis, SpO_2 < 92%, confusion
Circulation: pale, clammy, low blood pressure, faintness, drowsy/coma

---

[2] **Adrenaline** (give IM unless experienced with IV adrenaline)
IM doses of 1:1000 adrenaline (repeat after 5 min if no better)
- Adult   500 micrograms IM (0.5 mL)
- Child more than 12 years: 500 micrograms IM (0.5 mL)
- Child 6 -12 years: 300 micrograms IM (0.3 mL)
- Child less than 6 years: 150 micrograms IM (0.15 mL)

Adrenaline IV to be given **only by experienced specialists**
Titrate: Adults 50 micrograms; Children 1 microgram/kg

[3] **IV fluid challenge:**
Adult - 500 – 1000 mL
Child - crystalloid 20 mL/kg

Stop IV colloid
if this might be the cause
of anaphylaxis

---

	[4] **Chlorphenamine** (IM or slow IV)	[5] **Hydrocortisone** (IM or slow IV)
Adult or child more than 12 years	10 mg	200 mg
Child 6 - 12 years	5 mg	100 mg
Child 6 months to 6 years	2.5 mg	50 mg
Child less than 6 months	250 micrograms/kg	25 mg

March
2008

Figure 16.1 Management algorithm for anaphylaxis. (Reproduced with the kind permission of Resuscitation Council, UK.)

- EpiPen prescribed and educate the patient on administration and storage
- Medical alert bracelet

ACUTE ASTHMA

"A footballer with known asthma has been substituted late in the game for persistent cough and wheeze which is not responding to inhalers. His peak flow is 50% of his baseline. He is a known asthmatic with his last hospital admission 10 months ago. Please assess the player."

Asthma is a chronic respiratory disease characterised by airway inflammation, hyperresponsiveness and reversible obstruction.

The severity of asthma is summarised in Table 16.1.

Risk factors for severe asthma include:

- A previous intensive care unit (ITU) admission
- A recent attack within the past month, especially if oral steroids required
- ≥3 Accident and Emergency (A&E) attendances or ≥2 hospital admissions within the last year
- Lack of a written asthma action plan
- Socioeconomic problems, alcohol or substance abuse, mental health problems or non-concordance with treatment
- Comorbidities such as obesity, cardiovascular or chronic lung disease

Management of acute severe asthma:

1. ABCDE approach and call an ambulance
2. Give high flow oxygen 15 L/min via a non-rebreathe mask aiming for oxygen saturations $SaO_2 > 94\%$
3. Salbutamol 5 mg via oxygen-driven nebuliser – can give 'back to back'
4. Can add ipratropium 500 micrograms to nebuliser
5. Prednisolone 50 mg orally or hydrocortisone 200 mg IV

Monitor (if available): Oxygen saturations, arterial blood gas for the partial pressure of oxygen (PaO_2) and carbon dioxide ($PaCO_2$).

Re-review using ABCDE approach after every intervention given or change in patient's status.

These patients may require early intubation and will require hospital admission and ITU review.

On discharge and follow-up:

- Written asthma plan with own peak flow meter
- Education on inhaler technique
- GP follow-up within 2 days
- Follow-up in respiratory clinic within 4 weeks
- May be discharged with oral and inhaled steroids in addition to bronchodilators – may require a therapeutic use exemption (TUE)
- Athletes should not return to play until symptoms have completely resolved and peak flow is back to baseline. If in doubt or there are concerns about overall asthma control, seek advice from their respiratory physician

HYPOGLYCAEMIA

"A type 1 diabetic triathlete has just completed a morning training session and his teammates alert you to the fact that he is slurring his speech and appears confused."

Hypoglycaemia is a capillary blood glucose concentration <4.0 mmol/L, although some individuals may not show symptoms until blood sugar much lower than this.

Clinical features:

- Autonomic: Tremor, palpitations, anxiety, sweating, hunger
- Neuroglycopenic: Confusion, drowsiness, irritability, lethargy, irrational behaviour, seizure

Management:

1. ABCDE approach and full assessment including BM recording
2. Treat the hypoglycaemia (Table 16.2)
3. Recheck BM after 15 minutes
4. If able to swallow and BM > 4 mmol/L, give long-acting carbohydrates, e.g. biscuits, toast

Table 16.1 Clinical features of moderate, severe and life-threatening asthma

	Moderate asthma	Severe asthma	Life-threatening asthma
Clinical features or signs	• Increasing symptoms • PEFR > 50–75% best or predicted • No features of acute severe asthma	• PEFR 33–50% best or predicted • RR ≥ 25 breaths/min • HR ≥ 100 bpm • Unable to complete sentence in one breath	• Silent chest, cyanosis or feeble respiratory effort • Bradycardia or hypotension • Exhaustion or altered GCS • PEFR < 33% predicted or best • $SaO_2 < 92\%$

BPM, beats per minute; GCS, Glasgow Coma Scale; HR, heart rate; PEFR, peak flow; RR, respiratory rate; SaO₂, oxygen saturation

Table 16.2 Clinical features and recommended treatment in mild, moderate and severe hypoglycaemia

Severity	Mild	Moderate	Severe
Clinical features	Patient conscious, orientated and can swallow	Conscious but confused and able to swallow	Unconscious, seizing or very aggressive
Management	15–20 g of quick-acting carbohydrate, e.g. glucose tablets	1–2 tubes of glucose gel, e.g. Hypostop™	Glucose 1 mg IM or 10% glucose 100 mL/hr IV

IM, intramuscular; IV, intravenous.

Follow-up:

- Hypoglycaemia education
  - Check patient's understanding of hypo-glycaemia
  - Advise to monitor BMs before, during and after exercise
  - May require long-acting insulin adjust-ment (morning hypoglycaemic episodes may need evening insulin adjustment), training adjustment or greater carbohy-drate supplementation around training
  - Avoid exercise if BM > 14 mmol/L and/or ketones present
  - Carry a mobile and avoid exercising alone
- Refer to diabetic team if hypoglycaemia is unexplained, severe or recurrent
- May have to abstain from vigorous exercise for at least 24 hours due to possible delayed onset hypoglycaemia
- Note: Hypoglycaemia can occur in non-diabetic patients, especially with prolonged exercise or the following morning after excessive alcohol consumption
- In type 2 diabetics, sulfonylureas as well as insulin and to a lesser extent, meglitinides have the highest risk of hypoglycaemia with exercise

SEIZURES

Common causes:

- Hypoglycaemia
- Head injury
- Hypoxia
- Infection
- Intracranial pathology, e.g. space-occupying lesion (SOL), intracranial (IC) bleed
- Drugs
- Metabolic disturbance, e.g. hyponatraemia, hypocalcaemia
- Epilepsy

Management:

- Is it safe to approach?
- ABCDE approach and call for an ambulance
- Whilst having seizure:
  - High flow oxygen (15 L/min via non-rebreathe mask)

- Ensure the head is protected from harm and turn the patient semi-prone if not sus-pecting C-spine injury. Do not attempt to open the mouth
- If seizure is prolonged (>5 minutes) or repeated (3 or more in an hour), give diaze-pam 10 mg rectally or midazolam 10 mg buc-cal in adults (maximum 30 mg in 24 hours)
- Check for reversible causes if possible, e.g. BM, i-STAT for sodium
- Patient will require transfer to hospital for blood tests (full blood count [FBC], urea and electrolytes [U&E], liver function tests [LFTs], venous blood gas [VBG], drug screen), ECG and a computed tomography (CT) head scan
  - If this is the first presentation of a sei-zure, patient should be referred to first fit clinic on discharge – magnetic resonance imaging (MRI) head and electroencepha-logram (EEG) are normally organised by secondary care

Discharge and follow-up:

- Education: Advise the patient that there are not allowed to drive and that they will have to inform the Driver and Vehicle Licensing Agency (DVLA)
- No bathing with doors locked, showers are preferred to baths due to risk of submerging during washing
- Avoid dangerous sports where a seizure would put them at risk, e.g. rock climbing, abseiling
- There is little evidence that contact sports increase the risk of seizures but need to have sensible approach, especially if increased risk of head injury
- Ongoing individualised care plan will depend on underlying aetiology +/− liaising with the neurology team

HYPOTHERMIA

Hypothermia is present when core temperature is <35°C.

Mild: 32–35°C
Moderate: 29–32°C
Severe: <29°C

Clinical features:

- Mild: Lethargy, ataxia, shivering, tachypnoea
- Moderate: Bradycardia, hypotension, confusion, lack of shivering
- Severe: Coma, undetectable pulse, absent reflexes

Management:

- ABCDE approach and full assessment and call an ambulance
- Record the core temperature with a rectal thermometer
- Attempt to bring temperature up:
  Mild:
  - Remove any wet clothing and provide warm clothing or blankets
  - Rehydrate and give warm high-energy food and drink
  Moderate or severe:
  - Remove wet clothing and cover with warm blankets and/or emergency blanket
  - Give high flow oxygen (15 L/min via non-rebreathe mask)
  - Use air warming blanket, e.g. Bair Hugger® aiming for a core temperature rise of 1°C in young patients
  - Cautious warmed IV fluids if available
  - Prevent excessive movement as can precipitate ventricular fibrillation (VF)
  - If available, perform an ECG.

Possible ECG changes in hypothermia include bradyarrhythmias, J waves (positive deflection at the J point; Figure 16.2), prolonged PR interval, QRS or QT, shivering artefact and ventricular ectopics.

Changes to cardiac arrest algorithm if hypothermia:

- Pulse check for 1 min
- Double the interval of drugs if moderate (29–32°C)
- No drugs until >29°C
- VF shock ×3 then no more until core temperature >30°C
- Continue resuscitation attempts in hypothermia cardiac arrest until core temperature at least >33°C. This may require a prolonged period of resuscitation – *'you aren't dead until you are warm and dead'*

DROWNING

Drowning is a process that causes primary respiratory compromise following submersion (face and upper airway) or immersion (whole body) in water or another liquid.

Other factors to consider when assessing the drowning patient:

- Suspect cervical spine injury if diving involved
- Any preceding illness causing loss of consciousness (LOC) in water, e.g. arrhythmia
- Hypothermia
- Inhalation of contaminated water may require antibiotics

Management (Figure 16.3):

- Is it safe to approach?
- Call for help ask to ring ambulance
- Patient may need extrication from water with C-spine immobilisation in a horizontal position to prevent venous pooling

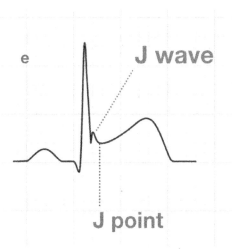

Figure 16.2 ECG depicting a typical J wave of hypothermia. (Image reproduced with kind permission from *Life in the Fast Lane* [https://litfl.com].)

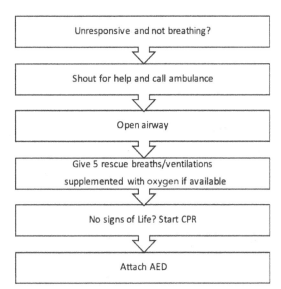

Figure 16.3 Algorithm for the management of drowning. (Abbreviations: CPR, cardiopulmonary resuscitation; AED, automatic external defibrillator.)

- Look, listen and feel once extricated from water
  - If in cardiac arrest, give five rescue breaths/ventilations – biggest cause of death is hypoxia, then start CPR 30:2
  - Dry off water before defibrillation
  - If concomitant hypothermia, may require prolonged CPR efforts
- If breathing with a pulse
  - ABCDE approach and assessment
  - Give high flow oxygen (15 L/min via a non-rebreathe mask)
  - May require suction of regurgitated stomach contents
  - Arrange transfer to hospital: common to have respiratory failure or acute respiratory distress syndrome (ARDS)

HYPERTHERMIA

Common causes of hyperthermia include:

- Hot weather
- Exercise
- Dermatological disease preventing heat dissipation, e.g. severe psoriasis
- Alcohol or illicit substances, e.g. cocaine and amphetamines
- Drugs, e.g. anticholinergics, inhaled general anaesthetics

Mild to moderate heat illness:

- Core temperature < 40°C
- Heat cramps
- Heat exhaustion: Thirst, headache, nausea and vomiting, flushed and sweating
- Tachycardia and orthostatic hypotension

Severe heat illness:

- Core temperature > 40°C and thermoregulatory mechanisms fail
- Exertional heat stroke is seen in young adults exercising in high ambient temperatures
- Headache, vomiting and diarrhoea, confusion, aggressive behaviour, collapse
- Hot dry skin, flushed
- Tachypnoeic, tachycardic and hypotensive
- Rhabdomyolysis, disseminated intravascular coagulation (DIC), multiorgan failure

Management:

If mild to moderate:
- Rest in a cool environment and cool them with soaked flannels and fanning
- Give up to 3 L cooled 0.9% NaCl (if no risk of hyponatraemia)
- May require admission for observation

Severe:
- Give high flow oxygen (15 L/min via non-rebreathe mask) aiming for SaO_2 >94%
- Urgent active cooling using wet flannels, fanning and ice packs to the groin and axilla aiming for core temperature <38.5°C
- Give 1 L cooled 0.9% NaCl (if no risk of hyponatraemia) then further according to BP and urine output
- May require benzodiazepines if seizures occur
- Measure and treat any concurrent hypoglycaemia
- Needs urgent transfer to hospital and ITU review

EXERCISE-ASSOCIATED HYPONATRAEMIA

"You are a doctor at the finish line medical tent at a marathon in southern Spain. An amateur runner crosses the finish line in 5 hours and collapses at the finish. They are noticeably bloated. Please assess."

Exercise-associated hyponatraemia (sodium [Na^+] < 135 mmol/L) has been documented in amateur runners who overhydrate with hypotonic fluids during endurance events (1). It may also be associated with a syndrome of inappropriate antidiuretic hormone secretion (SIADH) leading to water retention, which can exacerbate the clinical picture (2). It can be difficult to distinguish from other exertional illnesses such as heat stroke, so have a high index of suspicion in any exercise-associated collapse.

Clinical features:

- Nausea and vomiting
- Headache
- Dizziness
- Exhaustion and disorientation
- Muscle twitching
- Peripheral oedema
- Cardiovascular (CV) arrest or seizure

On clinical examination, assess for peripheral oedema, e.g. their wedding ring doesn't fit. Weighing the patient and comparing with their normal 'dry' weight if known can give a more accurate quantification of change.

Management:

Mild (Na^+ < 130 mmol/L)
- If normal GCS, then fluid restriction or oral hypertonic solutions

Moderate (Na^+ 125–129 mmol/L) to Severe (Na^+ < 125 mmol/L)
- Fluid restrict
- Catheterise to monitor accurate urine input and output

- Give hypertonic 3% NaCl 100 mL/hr until levels between 128–130 mmol/L (can repeat every 10 minutes)
- Daily weight
- Admission to hospital

All patients require education about appropriate hydration during exercise to *'drink to thirst'*.

Note: A too rapid correction of hyponatraemia (>6 mmol/L) may cause coma associated with osmotic demyelination syndrome or central pontine demyelinosis.

AUTONOMIC DYSREFLEXIA IN PARA-ATHLETES

This is a common scenario and an important medical emergency in athletes with a spinal cord injury that is easy to examine in OSCEs. Potential scenarios could include managing someone in an acute crisis or explaining to an athlete the diagnosis and signs and symptoms to look out for.

"Steve is a 34-year-old paraplegic wheelchair racer (with a T4 cord resection) due to race in 2 days. You are travelling on the team coach with him and the rest of the team and another athlete comes to notify you that Steve is clammy and flushed and complaining of a headache. Please clinically assess him."

"A wheelchair basketballer had an episode of autonomic dysreflexia last month, assumed to be triggered by a pressure sore. She has come to see you as at the time she did not fully understand what happened and would like to discuss ongoing management and prevention."

Autonomic dysreflexia is an unregulated sympathetic drive from a noxious stimulus in anyone with a spinal cord lesion at **T6 or above**. Systemic vasoconstriction is normally countered by vasodilation of the splanchnic vascular bed to reduce blood pressure. As the splanchnic bed receives innervation from T5–T9, lesions of the spinal cord above this level allow uninhibited sympathetic tone as descending inhibitory parasympathetic signals are blocked, causing dangerous hypertension. It is common in those with catheters. If left unmanaged, it can result in myocardial infarction, intracranial haemorrhage, or death.

Causes:
The 6 B's: Bladder, Bowel, Back passage, Boils, Babies (3)
- Bladder distension (75–85% of cases)
- Urinary tract infection (UTI)
- Bowel impaction
- Deep vein thrombosis (DVT)
- Ingrown toenail
- Pressure ulcer
- Obstetric

Table 16.3 Clinical features of autonomic dysreflexia

Above the injury (parasympathetic response)	Below the injury (sympathetic response)
• Headache and flushing • Sweating • Bradycardia • Pupillary constriction • Nasal congestion • Blurred vision • Anxiety	Pale, cool skin Piloerection (goose bumps)
Significant rise in systolic and diastolic BP greater than 20 mmHg systolic or 10 mmHg diastolic above baseline – remember spinal cord injury patients normally have a low systolic BP (SBP).	

Signs and Symptoms: Signs and symptoms are summarised in Table 16.3. Suspect the diagnosis in any patient with a spinal cord injury at level T6 or above with a headache.

Clinical assessment of the patient:

- Perform an ABCDE assessment
- Take a brief clinical history and specifically ask about some of the symptoms above, in particular, catheter care or when last opened/evacuated bowels. Establish if they are on any medication or have any allergies
- Check the observations including blood pressure
  - If this is raised, immediately sit the patient up and loosen their clothing (to allow for lower extremity pooling of blood)
- Briefly assess cranial nerves for pupillary constriction and vision and comment on any of the signs and symptoms mentioned above
- Next, try to ascertain and treat the cause (as removing this should restore BP)
  - Given it is the most common cause, start with urinary system – if they are catheterised, check along its entire length for kinks, constrictions or obstruction and correct placement. If it appears blocked, say you would irrigate with normal saline. If they are not catheterised, consider doing so
  - If catheter not blocked, suspect fecal impaction – say you would perform a per rectum (PR) examination to assess for fecal impaction. If there is impaction, state you would treat this with manual evacuation/enema and laxative
  - Check feet and skin on the lower half of body for pressure sores or ingrown toenails

- If you have been able to remedy the cause, continue to monitor BP and pulse every 2–5 minutes until stabilised (fluctuations are common though)
  - If BP does not return to baseline within 5–10 minutes or the SBP is >150 mmHg, begin medical treatment (3)
- If no cause found, consider use of fast-acting antihypertensive if SBP > 150 mmHg. Repeat doses every 20–30 minutes as required
  - Nifedipine 5–10 mg orally or sublingual
  - GTN 2 puffs sublingual
  - GTN patch 0.2 mg/hr above level of lesion
- Caution in patients also on Sildenafil as nitrates are contraindicated here
- Monitor BP for at least 2 hours after episode to ensure no rebound hypotension

Aftercare:

- Educate patient regarding prevention, e.g. regular catheter drainage
- Warn recurrent attacks can occur up to 10 days after
- Supply medical alert bracelet
- Supply with small supply of nifedipine to have on them at all times
- May need to contact specialist spinal rehabilitation team if no obvious trigger or recurrent episodes for further investigations, e.g. bladder and bowel assessment

Clinical pearls:

- Sit the patient up and take a blood pressure reading early
- Try to identify and rectify the causative issue
- Strongly suspect this diagnosis in patients with spinal cord injury at T6 or above with a headache

Things to avoid:

- Not sitting patient up
- Giving medication before assessment of cause (as this should restore BP if reversed)
- Not providing a safe aftercare plan
- If giving an explanation to patient, using too much medical jargon

CARDIOPULMONARY RESUSCITATION

Cardiopulmonary resuscitation is required if a collapsed person is unresponsive, not breathing and has no palpable central pulse, e.g. carotid or femoral.

The adult Advanced Life Support algorithm is shown in Figure 16.4.

Management:

- Is it safe to approach?
- Is patient responding?

- If no response, look, listen and feel for 10 seconds (look at chest wall, listen for breathing and feel for breath sounds against your face) whilst simultaneously feeling carotid pulse. Ideally, this should be whilst doing a head tilt, chin lift
- If no signs of life, call for help and start chest compressions
  - Heel of hand in centre of the chest, compressions at a depth of 5–6 cm at a rate of 100 compressions/minute, allowing for recoil between compressions
  - Ratio of 30:2 compressions: ventilations with a bag valve mask
- When help arrives, ask them to call for an ambulance and to bring back a defibrillator with them. If you are alone, say you would call for an ambulance then return to commence CPR
- As soon as defibrillator arrives, apply self-adhesive pads whilst continuing chest compressions and analyse the rhythm with a brief pause in chest compressions. Some automated external defibrillators (AEDs) will not require manual analysis of the rhythm and will charge or not accordingly

Shockable rhythms: VF or ventricular tachycardia (VT)

Non-shockable rhythms: Pulseless electrical activity (PEA) or asystole

- If a **shockable rhythm**, charge the defibrillator, continuing chest compressions whilst charging (this is to minimise time off the chest, but some AEDs may instruct to stop compressions whilst charging)
- Ensure all individuals clear and oxygen moved then deliver a 150–200 J direct current (DC) shock via a biphasic waveform defibrillator and *immediately* resume chest compressions
- Continue chest compressions at 30:2 for 2 minutes, then briefly pause to assess rhythm again
- Meanwhile, establish an intravenous line in a central vein to deliver medications
- If VF/VT remains, give a second DC shock of 150–360 J biphasic, recommence CPR and reassess after 2 mins
- If VF/VT remains, give a third shock of 150–360 J biphasic, recommence CPR and give:
  - 1 mg of 1 in 10,000 adrenaline IV
  - 300 mg amiodarone IV
  - Irrespective of arrest rhythm given additional 1 mg of 1 in 10,000 adrenaline IV every other cycle (every 3–5 minutes)
- You can also give a further 150 mg of amiodarone after the 5th shock

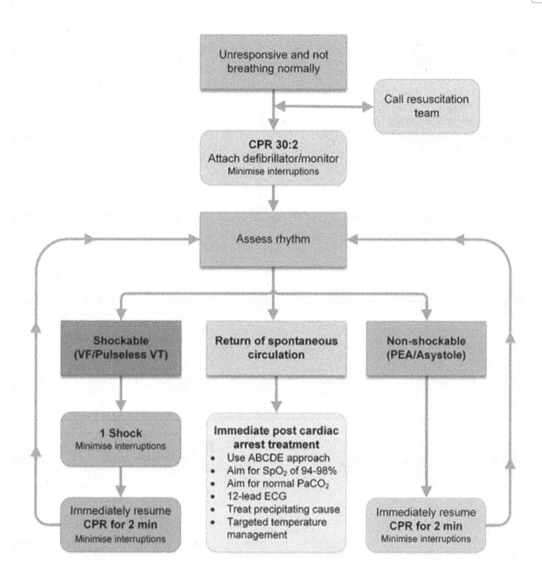

Figure 16.4 Adult advanced life support (ALS) algorithm. (Reproduced with the kind permission of Resuscitation Council, UK.)

- If a **non-shockable** rhythm, continue CPR with reassessment of rhythm and pulse every 2 minutes and establish an intravenous line and give 1 mg of 1 in 10,000 adrenaline as soon as possible, and then every other cycle (3–5 minutes)
- In all cases, identify any potentially reversible causes the '4 H's and the 4 T's'. Try to address these and name them out loud, e.g. check core temperature, ensure 100% oxygen

  - Hypoxia
  - Hypovolaemia
  - Hypo-/hyperkalaemia/metabolic
  - Hypothermia

- Thrombosis – coronary or pulmonary
- Tension pneumothorax
- Tamponade – cardiac
- Toxins

If at any point there are signs of life suggesting return of spontaneous circulation (ROSC), then begin post-resuscitation care. Patient will require admission to the hospital and ITU review with further investigations.

REFERENCES

1. Rosner MH, Kirven J. Exercise-associated hyponatremia. *Clin J Am Soc Nephrol.* 2007;2:151–61.
2. Hew-Butler T, Dugas JP, Noakes TD, Verbalis JG. Changes in plasma arginine vasopressin concentrations in cyclists participating in a 109-km cycle race. *Br J Sports Med.* 2010;44:594–7.
3. Cowan H, Lakra C, Desai M. Autonomic dysreflexia in spinal cord injury. *BMJ.* 2020;371:m3596.

17 Trauma

INTRODUCTION

The assessment and management of a patient with acute trauma is a common acute scenario that can be easily examined in sports and exercise medicine (SEM) objective structured clinical examinations (OSCEs). It is likely that these types of scenarios will be in a pre-hospital or pitch-side setting. Similar to medical emergencies, simulation training is invaluable in preparing you for the steps to undertake to carry out a timely and safe assessment of patients with trauma. Ensure you are aware of the up-to-date guidance on head injuries and indications for referral to secondary care for any type of traumatic injury.

HEAD INJURY

Head injuries can range from concussion/mild traumatic brain injury to a more serious injury requiring further investigations and imaging. You need to be familiar with the guidelines and the sport and environment you are working in, e.g. whether off-field screening tools are being used such as the Head Injury Assessment (HIA) protocol (1), or whether the instructions for head injuries is to 'recognise and remove'.

Signs and symptoms of concussion/mild traumatic brain injury either witnessed or observed on video include, but are not limited to:

Signs:

- Loss of consciousness (LOC)
- Blank or vacant look
- Disorientation or confusion or inability to respond appropriately to questions
- Ataxia/gait difficulties/motor incoordination or slow, laboured movement
- Facial injury after head trauma

Symptoms:

- Headache
- Dizziness
- Nausea or vomiting
- Blurred vision
- Feeling 'in a fog'
- Confusion
- Irritability
- Emotional
- Difficulty concentrating or remembering
- Balance problems

On-field indications for **permanent** removal of play:

1. Definite LOC
2. Suspected LOC
3. Ataxia
4. Seizure
5. Oculomotor signs
6. Tonic posturing
7. Confusion
8. Disorientated in time, place or person
9. Clearly dazed
10. Definite behaviour change
11. On-field sign or symptoms of concussion
12. Doctor decision

Indications for off-field screening, e.g. HIA if resources available:

- Head injury where diagnosis not apparent
- Possible behaviour change or possible confusion
- Injury event witnessed with potential to result in concussive injury

If permanently replaced, then go on to perform:

- Secondary survey
- Clinical assessment using the Sport Assessment Concussion Tool (SCAT5) (2)
- Regular monitoring
- Provide concussion advice
  - Not to be left alone for 48 hours
  - Not to drive or drink alcohol
  - Appropriate transport home
  - Suitable follow-up plan

DOI: 10.1201/9781003163701-21

Indications for referral to A&E with a head injury (National Institute for Health and Care Excellence [NICE] guidelines) for computed tomography (CT) scan of the head are shown in Figure 17.1 (3).

- Patients will require a CT scan of their head with any of the following **within 1 hour**:
  - Glasgow Coma Scale (GCS) < 13
  - GCS < 15 at 2 hours
  - Open or depressed skull fracture
  - Sign of base of skull fracture
  - Post-traumatic seizure
- Focal neurological deficit
- >1 episode of vomiting
- Amnesia > 30 minutes before impact
- Patients will require a CT scan of their head if they have experienced loss of consciousness or amnesia AND any of the following **within 8 hours**:
  - Age > 65 years
  - Dangerous mechanism of injury (MOI)
  - History of bleeding or clotting disorders
  - 30 minutes retrograde amnesia of events

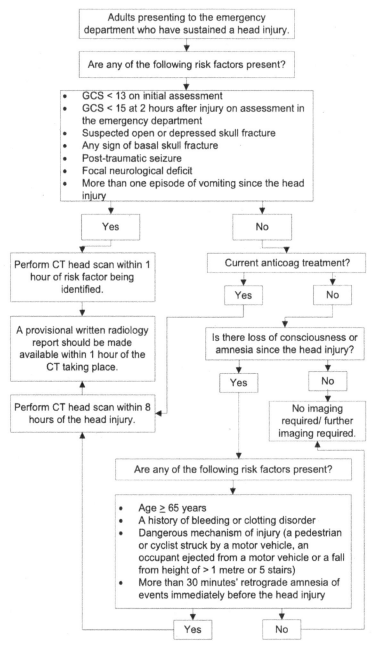

Figure 17.1 NICE Guidance on indications for CT head in adults. (Reproduced from *Head Injury* [2014], Clinical Guideline 176, published by the National Guideline Centre at the Royal College of Physicians, 11 St Andrews Place, Regent's Park, London, NW11 4LE. Copyright © NGC. Reproduced by permission.)

- Patients will require a CT scan of their head within 8 hours if they are on warfarin

Dangerous MOI include the following:

- Fall from >1 metre or 5 stairs
- Axial load to head
- High-speed motor vehicle collision
- Rollover motor vehicle accident
- Ejection from motor vehicle
- Accident involving motorised recreational vehicles
- Bicycle collision

CLEARING THE CERVICAL SPINE

This is a skill which should be practiced and that has previously come up as an assessed element in pitch-side OSCE stations. You should be familiar with a validated criteria to clear the cervical spine, e.g. National Emergency X-Radiography Utilisation Group (NEXUS) criteria (4) or Canadian C-spine rules (5) and understand how to put them into practice in a clinical case.

You cannot clear the cervical spine if any of the following are present:

- Dangerous mechanism of injury (as above)
- Pain in the cervical spine
- Pain on palpation of the cervical spine
- Traumatic brain injury and/or skull fracture
- Under the influence of alcohol or drugs
- Has any significant distracting injuries
- Has a reduced level of consciousness
- Is confused or uncooperative
- Has any hand or foot weakness (motor)
- Has altered or absent sensation in the hands or feet (sensory)
- Has a past history of spinal problems

"You are covering a lacrosse game in which a 25-year-old player has had a heavy collision with another player. There is no suspicion of axial loading or another high-risk mechanism of injury. You have performed a full ABCDE assessment on the pitch but due to the player being dazed at the time, they have been extricated to the medical room for further assessment. The player is now alert. Please could you reassess the player and explain and demonstrate how you would clear their cervical spine."

1. Repeat the ABCDE assessment now the patient has been moved, as above
2. If using NEXUS criteria, ensure:
   a. Normal alertness (A on AVPU or GCS 15)
   b. No intoxication
   c. No painful distracting injury
3. Palpate posterior midline cervical spine for tenderness
4. Assess for any focal neurological deficit – examine torso, legs and arms for motor and/or sensory deficits

5. If it satisfies all of the above:
   a. Explain to the patient what you would like to do with clear instructions
   b. Warn the patient that if at any point there is pain, neurological symptoms, e.g. tingling or a block, stop movement, ask them to return to the midline and replace collar
   c. Carefully remove collar whilst having patient keep their head still
   d. Have the patient move their head 45° left and right
   e. Have the patient flex and extend their head
6. If the patient can perform above, then carefully sit up and ask them to perform the movements again sitting up

Note: NEXUS criteria have 99.6% sensitivity but may not be reliable in patients >65 years.

If following the Canadian C-spine rules:

Assess whether the person is at high, low or no risk for cervical spine injury using the Canadian C-spine rules as follows:

The person is at high risk if they have at least one of the following high-risk factors:

1. Age 65 years or older
2. Dangerous mechanism of injury (detailed above)
3. Paraesthesia in the upper or lower limbs

The person is at low risk if they have at least one of the following low-risk factors:

- Involved in a minor rear-end motor vehicle collision
- Comfortable in a sitting position
- Ambulatory at any time since the injury
- No midline cervical spine tenderness
- Delayed onset of neck pain

The person remains at low risk if they are:

- Able to actively rotate their neck 45° to the left and right (the range of the neck can only be assessed safely if the person is at low risk and there are no high-risk factors)

No radiography required if they:

- Have one of the above low-risk factors and
- Are able to actively rotate their neck 45° to the left and right

Imaging is required for any high risk criteria, anyone who doesn't satisfy any of the low-risk criteria or is unable to rotate their neck 45° to the left and right.

Note in cases of 'stingers', i.e. a transient brachial plexus neuropraxia, symptoms should be unilateral, players should have no pain or symptoms in the neck, and symptoms should fully resolve within a few minutes. Players should not be allowed to return to play if any deficits present. If at any point symptoms are bilateral or symptoms are prolonged, then follow the cervical spine guidance as above.

Caution in players who have 'recurrent' stingers (>2 episodes); they may require further imaging to assess for stenosis or other structural abnormalities.

FACIAL TRAUMA

Zygomatic complex fracture

"A 35-year-old hockey player has taken a blow to the side of his face and has walked off the pitch and is now in the medical room. You have done a full A-E assessment which is satisfactory. He is clutching his right cheek which is swollen but is sitting up and is alert and orientated. Please take a focussed history and examination and explain your management."

Focussed history:

- Mechanism of injury
- Concussion symptoms
- Ask about vision
- Nose – can they breathe through both nostrils?
- Teeth – any paraesthesia or pain in their teeth or mouth?
- Zygoma – any pain or deformity?
- SCAT5

Examination:

From front:

Inspection – swelling or lacerations, tooth avulsions

Full cranial nerve examination but specifically examine:

- Vision
  - Assess acuity using Snellen chart or count fingers
  - Eye movements and ask if diplopia – **note orbital floor 'blow-out' fractures can tether the inferior rectus muscle causing diplopia on downgaze or difficulty with upgaze**
    - Requires facial X-ray or CT scan – look for opaque maxillary sinus or a fluid level from bleeding and a 'tear-drop' soft-tissue opacity hanging from the roof of the sinus
  - Visual fields
  - Pupillary reflex
- Sensation – Trigeminal (V) nerve
  - Forehead – supraorbital nerve
  - Cheek – infraorbital nerve (also innervates top teeth)
  - Lower lip – mental nerve
- Facial movements - Facial (VII) nerve
  - Wounds in parotid area risk damaging the facial nerve

Mandible occlusion – ask to clench teeth and ask if it feels normal

Check for sublingual haematoma. Mandible fracture unlikely if bite feels normal, can open mouth against resistance and no tenderness when both mamdible angles compressed.

- Inspect inside the mouth and ask to bite down – look for steps or gaping in teeth
- Le Fort fractures: Medial and lateral buttress tenderness – test stability

Orbits – palpate around supra and infraorbital rim. Subcutaneous emphysema indicates possible maxillary sinus fracture

Zygoma – palpate for bony tenderness and assess for flattening of the cheekbone

Nose – palpate and look for septal haematoma – a septal haematoma **requires drainage to prevent saddle nose deformity**

Skull – palpate for any boggy swellings

Neck – palpate for swelling, tenderness or crepitus

Other: Check for cerebrospinal fluid (CSF) leak from nose or ears, check for Battle's sign and raccoon eyes indicating the base of skull fracture

From behind, looking down face from above:

Inspection – assess for enophthalmos for orbital floor fracture and zygoma asymmetry

Management for suspected zygomatic complex fracture:

- ABCDE
- Analgesia
- Refer to hospital with maxillofacial unit for further assessment including X-rays with occipitomental views and/or CT
- Tell patient not to blow nose as subcutaneous emphysema may result if paranasal sinuses involved
- Urgent maxillofacial referral for consideration of closed or open reduction if fracture
- Follow-up the patient for assessment and management of concomitant concussion

The following suspected injuries require urgent referral to hospital:

- Zygomaticomaxillary complex fractures
- Fractured or dislocated mandible
- Le Fort fractures
- Dental: Avulsed tooth. Ask the player to put in buccal fold, milk or saline in meantime
- Full thickness of lip lacerations which breach the vermilion border
- Ophthalmic:
  - Orbital floor fracture, globe rupture, retinal detachment, lens dislocation, hyphema
  - Blurred vision or diplopia, photophobia, flashing lights, reduced visual acuity, loss of visual field, unable to tolerate the exam

Familiarise yourself with appropriate management for common traumatic eye injuries and dental problems.

Acute epistaxis

"A hockey player has taken a direct blow to the face from another player and is kneeling on the pitch clutching their nose which is bleeding profusely. You are the doctor pitch-side and first to assess the patient."

Management of acute epistaxis:

- Is it safe to approach?
- On pitch ABCDE assessment
- If the patient is haemodynamically compromised, perform measures to stem bleeding +/− IV cannulation and IV fluid resuscitation
  - Sit the patient up with their upper body tilted forward and their mouth open
  - Pinch the anterior cartilaginous part of the nose firmly and hold it for 10 minutes and ask them to breathe through their mouth until bleeding stops
  - Forbid the patient to pick, blow or sniff through the nose to prevent recurrence
  - If bleeding does not stop after 10–15 minutes of nasal pressure, if trained, can attempt:
    - Nasal cautery of the bleeding point with a silver nitrate stick touched onto the area for <10 seconds
    - Anterior nasal tamponade by inserting a nasal tampon, e.g. Merocel® or inflatable packs, e.g. Rapid-Rhino®. Secure the pack and ensure there is no pressure on the cartilage around the nostril
- If haemostasis cannot be achieved in the pre-hospital setting, then admit the patient to hospital for observation via ear, nose and throat (ENT) team for secondary care treatments
- Palpate and look for septal haematoma – a septal haematoma requires drainage to prevent saddle nose deformity. Deviated fractures can be reduced immediately or be sent to Accident and Emergency (A&E)

Advice for the 24 hours following acute epistaxis episode include avoiding:

- Blowing or picking the nose
- Heavy lifting
- Strenuous exercise
- Lying flat
- Drinking alcohol or hot drinks

CHEST TRAUMA

TENSION PNEUMOTHORAX

A tension pneumothorax is characterised by positive pressure exerted on mediastinal and intrathoracic structures due to a progressive accumulation of intrapleural air. It can, therefore, potentially lead to life-threatening cardiorespiratory compromise.

Clinical features:

- Respiratory distress
- Chest pain
- Ipsilateral reduced expansion
- Ipsilateral reduced breath sounds
- Hyperresonant on percussion
- Tachypnoea and tachycardia
- Agitation
- Late: Hypotension, reduced GCS, tracheal deviation, distended neck veins

Management:

- ABCDE approach and call for ambulance
- High flow oxygen (15 L/min via non-rebreathe mask)
- Immediate decompression via needle thoracocentesis
  - Wide bore cannula
  - Second intercostal space, midclavicular line – should hear hiss of air
  - Alternative if large pectoralis major: fifth intercostal space just anterior to mid axillary line
  - Reassess after intervention
- Transfer to hospital for definitive chest drain and imaging

MASSIVE HAEMOTHORAX

A massive haemothorax is the rapid accumulation of blood >1500 mL or one-third of the blood volume in the chest cavity.

Clinical features:

- Tachycardia +/− hypotension
- Ipsilateral dullness to percussion
- Ipsilateral reduced breath sounds
- Dyspnoea
- Anxiety or confusion

Management:

- ABCDE
- High flow oxygen (15 L/min via non-rebreathe mask)
- Gain IV access using at least one large bore cannula (16g) in large vein
  - If unable, then use intraosseous (IO) needle at proximal tibia, distal tibia or proximal humerus
- Fluid resuscitation with crystalloid if radial pulse lost* (blood is normally not available in pre-hospital setting)

*Note: Do not fluid resuscitate in trauma setting if radial pulse is present to avoid disrupting the initial clot – *'the first clot is the best clot'*.

- Urgent transfer to trauma centre for definitive management: Imaging, chest drain, IV fluids +/− thoracotomy

ABDOMINAL TRAUMA

SPLENIC INJURY

Blunt abdominal trauma causing lower left rib injuries can cause splenic injuries. Splenic rupture can also occur without rib fracture and in cases where individuals already have an enlarged spleen, e.g. Glandular fever (Epstein-Barr virus [EBV]).

The clinical features are summarised in Table 17.1

Management:

- ABCDE approach
- High flow oxygen (15 L/min via non-rebreathe mask)
- Gain IV access using at least one large bore cannula (16g) in large vein
  - If unable, then use intraosseous needle at proximal tibia, distal tibia or proximal humerus
- Fluid resuscitation with crystalloid if radial pulse lost (blood is normally not available in pre-hospital setting)
- Urgent transfer to trauma centre for definitive management: Imaging and laparotomy

MUSCULOSKELETAL TRAUMA

PELVIC INJURY

The major complication of pelvic fracture is massive blood loss, which may not be immediately obvious. They normally result from high-energy blunt trauma such as a fall from height. Associated bladder, urethral, rectal and vaginal injuries can occur.

Clinical features:

- Pain in the groin, hip or lower back
- Pain worse on moving legs/inability to weight bear
- Swelling of the pelvic area
- Uneven leg length or asymmetry of iliac wings
- Numbness or tingling in the perineum or top of the thigh
- Perineal ecchymoses, scrotal or labial haematomas

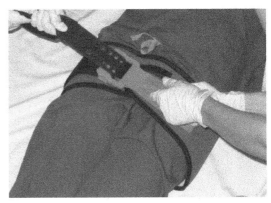

Figure 17.2 Placement of a pelvic binder, e.g. SAM Sling™ ratched compression belt requires two people and should be placed at the level of the greater trochanters. (Reproduced with kind permission from *Apley & Solomon's System of Orthopaedics and Trauma*, 10th edition, CRC Press, 2018.)

- Blood from the urethral meatus

Management:

- ABCDE approach and call an ambulance
- High flow oxygen (15 L/min via non-rebreathe mask)
- Gain IV access using at least one large bore cannula (16g) in large vein
  - If unable, then use intraosseous needle at proximal tibia, distal tibia or proximal humerus
- Fluid resuscitation with small bolus of crystalloid if radial pulse lost
- Stabilise the pelvis
  - Bring knees, ankles and toes together
  - Place pelvic binder using a second person at level of greater trochanters (Figure 17.2)
  - Assess for pulses before and after applying the binder. If pulses lost on application of the binder, do not reattempt to reposition the binder.
  - Avoid compression and distraction of the pelvis or excessive log-rolling if possible
- Urgent transfer to trauma centre for definitive management

Table 17.1 Acute and delayed clinical features of splenic injury	
Acute	**Delayed (up to 2 weeks)**
• Tachycardia and hypotension • Abdominal tenderness • Shoulder-tip pain (referred) • Localised pain – lower left rib	• Localised pain • Shoulder-tip pain
Source: Adapted from *Apley & Solomon's System of Orthopaedics and Trauma*, 10th edition, CRC Press (2018).	

Note: Do not remove a pelvic binder until it is radiologically confirmed that there is no fracture present.

LIMB INJURY

Clinical features:

- Obvious deformity, tenderness or swelling
- Localised pain
- Neurovascular compromise: Diminished pulses, discolouration, cool skin
- Crepitus and tenderness
- Features of compartment syndrome
- Assess for fractures threatening the viability of the skin

Head, thoracic, abdominal and pelvic injuries would normally take priority over limb injuries.

Management:

- ABCDE and call for ambulance
- High flow oxygen (15 L/min via non-rebreathe mask)
- Gain IV access if likely extensive haemorrhage using at least one large bore cannula (16g) in large vein
  - If unable, then use intraosseous needle at proximal tibia, distal tibia or proximal humerus different to the site of limb injury, e.g. contralateral limb. Cannot use if there is a fracture proximal to insertion site or if any previous IO inserted proximally has tissued
- Fluid resuscitation with crystalloid using small boluses if radial pulse lost (blood is normally not available in pre-hospital setting)
- Assess for neurological deficit, e.g. radial nerve damage in humeral shaft fracture
- Assess for vascular compromise by palpating pulses and assessing temperature
- Open wounds should be irrigated with copious amounts of 0.9% saline
- Open fractures should be covered with a saline-soaked sterile dressing (these should not be irrigated in the pre-hospital setting) and antibiotics administered intravenously as soon as an open fracture is identified, ideally within 1 hour of the injury
- Restore deformity to normal anatomical alignment and recheck pulses. If possible, give appropriate analgesia during, e.g. Entonox (50% nitrous oxide and 50% oxygen) or Penthrox (methoxyflurane) if no contraindications (see the box titled 'Contraindications to Entonox and Penthrox®')

Contraindications to Entonox and Penthrox

Contraindications to Entonox

- Head injuries and reduced GCS
- Chest injuries
- Air embolism
- Maxillofacial injuries
- Decompression sickness
- Intoxication

Contraindications to Penthrox

- Head injuries and reduced GCS
- Hepatorenal disease
- Aged <18 years
- Any previous reaction to anaesthetic agents

Restoring normal anatomical alignment will:

- Reduce pain
- Reduce the risk of neurovascular compromise
- Maintain skin integrity

Some will advocate returning limb back to original position if reduction causes loss of pulse and recheck for reappearance of pulses.

- Immobilise the fracture using suitable splint covering joint above and below, e.g. box splint. Recheck pulses after splinting
- Transfer to trauma centre for definitive management

Other notes: If available, give flucloxacillin 2 g IV and tetanus prophylaxis.

REFERENCES

1. Fuller CW, Fuller GW, Kemp SP, Raftery M. Evaluation of world Rugby's concussion management process: Results from Rugby World Cup 2015. *Br J Sports Med*. 2017;51: 64–9.
2. Echemendia RJ, Meeuwisse W, McCrory P. Sport concussion assessment tool, 5th edition. *Br J Sports Med*. 2017;51:851–8.
3. NICE NIfHaCE. *Head Injury*. London: National Clinical Guideline Centre; 2014.
4. Hoffman JR, Mower WR, Wolfson AB, Todd KH, Zucker MI. Validity of a set of clinical criteria to rule out injury to the cervical spine in patients with blunt trauma. National Emergency X-Radiography Utilization Study Group. *N Engl J Med*. 2000;343(2):94–9.
5. Stiell IG, Wells GA, Vandemheen KL, Clement CM, Lesiuk H, De Maio VJ, et al. The Canadian C-spine rule for radiography in alert and stable trauma patients. *JAMA*. 2001;286:1841–8.

18 Radiology

Natalie F. Shur & Arieff Abuhassan, Consultant Musculoskeletal Radiologist, Nottingham University Hospitals NHS Trust

INTRODUCTION

Selection of an appropriate imaging modality and interpretation of radiological images are key skills for a sport and exercise medicine physician in both confirming an accurate diagnosis and in management planning. In the context of a Sport and Exercise Medicine (SEM) objective structured clinical examination (OSCE), it is unlikely that a station will be devoted entirely to image interpretation, but single images have appeared within clinical stations previously. This chapter will cover some of the basic principles of radiology in the context of Sport and Exercise Medicine and then detail the key features of important diagnoses that you should be familiar with. Regular attendance at radiology meetings and assessing and discussing scans with colleagues at every opportunity will improve your knowledge and ability to read scans.

BASICS OF MUSCULOSKELETAL RADIOLOGY

IMAGING MODALITIES

Common imaging modalities used in musculoskeletal medicine are shown in Table 18.1. Other modalities include nuclear medicine specialised scans, MR or computed tomography (CT) arthrogram for labral injuries (glenohumeral or hip) and MR arthrogram for diagnosis of injuries to the triangular fibrocartilage complex (TFCC).

HOW TO INTERPRET AN X-RAY

Have an organised, systematic approach to review any image, e.g. ABC'S (see following text). Another sequence is "the patient, the soft tissues, the bones, the joints."

DOI: 10.1201/9781003163701-22

Table 18.1 Imaging modalities commonly used in the evaluation of the musculoskeletal system and sports injuries

Modality	Application
X-ray	• First-line inexpensive modality for localised evaluation of musculoskeletal pain • Can detect acute bony or joint fractures or dislocations • Can detect calcification • May miss subtle or occult disease • Poor soft-tissue contrast • Exposure to ionising radiation
Ultrasound (US)	• No radiation risk, quick, cheap and readily available • Accuracy depends on operator expertise • Diagnostic or therapeutic procedures, e.g. joint aspiration • Dynamic evaluation possible • Multiplanar imaging • Doppler ultrasound can be useful in suspected inflammation
Computed tomography (CT)	• Excellent for bony trauma or abnormalities • Quicker than magnetic resonance imaging (MRI) • Cross-sectional imaging with multiplanar reformats • Good for complex joints • Axial structures • Excellent contrast resolution and spatial localisation • Higher radiation exposure than plain radiographs • Poor soft-tissue contrast compared with MRI
Magnetic resonance imaging (MRI)	• Excellent soft-tissue contrast • No radiation risk • Currently, there is an unknown risk from gadolinium contrast tissue deposition • Cross-sectional imaging • Contraindicated with some pacemakers, implants and history of metallic foreign bodies • Patients may not tolerate (e.g. claustrophobia) • Expensive • Studies may take up to an hour (e.g. whole body MRI)

- Anatomy, Alignment and joint space – look for changes in alignment indicating a fracture, subluxation or dislocation, joint space narrowing or osteophyte formation or subchondral sclerosis
- Bone texture – a change in density within the matrix or cortex can indicate pathology
- Cortex and cartilage – a fracture in the cortex may be identified as a step, lucency or sclerosis, or in paediatric patients, the cortex may remain smooth (the 'greenstick' fracture). A periosteal reaction can occur in response to injury, infection or malignancy but is not present in the acute setting
- Soft tissues – assess for soft-tissue swelling or effusions

HOW TO PRESENT AN X-RAY

- Open with a description of film and orientate yourself with the view (Figure 18.1), e.g. 'this is an anteroposterior (AP) plain film of a knee joint in an adult patient'
- Comment on adequacy – rotation, penetration, expansion
- Describe the main abnormality
- Review other areas and comment
- Compare with previous imaging
- Offer the diagnosis and any relevant differentials

How to report a fracture:

1. Describe the film
   - What type of radiograph are you looking at?
   - What views do you have, e.g. frontal (AP) or lateral?

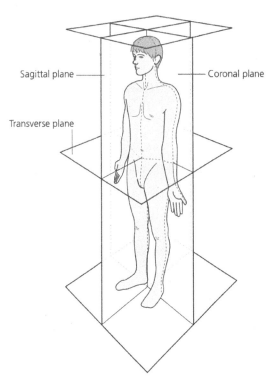

Figure 18.1 The principal planes of the body, as viewed in the anatomical position: Sagittal, coronal and transverse (axial). (Reproduced with kind permission from *Apley & Solomon's System of Orthopaedics and Trauma*, 10th edition, CRC Press, 2018.)

Sagittal plane

Coronal plane

Transverse plane

2. Fracture type
   • Complete (transverse, oblique, spiral, comminuted)
   • Incomplete (buckle, greenstick)
3. Fracture location
   • Which bone
   • Part of the bone (epiphysis, metaphysis, diaphysis, apophysis)
4. Fracture displacement
   • Described in terms of the distal fragment to the body
   • Angulation, translation or rotation
5. Fracture complications
   • Evidence of compound fracture (through the skin)
   • Does the fracture enter the joint
   • Is there another fracture (e.g. in paired bones)

Patterns of abnormalities are important to make a diagnosis. If you see one abnormality that is suggestive, look for others that are associated.

• Joint space narrowing, subchondral sclerosis and cysts and osteophytes = osteoarthritis

• Joint space narrowing, osteoporosis and periarticular erosions = inflammatory arthritis. If symmetrical polyarthropathy of the proximal joints of the hands, think rheumatoid arthritis
• Bone destruction and periosteal new bone formation = infection or malignancy until proven otherwise

MRI FOR SPORT AND EXERCISE MEDICINE

MRI is a commonly used modality in SEM and an understanding of the basic physics of MRI is important to appreciate the differences in sequences and to interpret the findings in front of you. The patient is placed in a magnetic field produced within the MRI scanner which aligns the positively charged protons in the body, known as 'spins'. Spins are perturbed by radiofrequency (RF) pulses and as they realign with the magnetic field, will produce a signal which is detected by the scanner. The amount of time between successive pulse sequences applied to the same slide is known as the repetition time (TR). The speed of tissue relaxation combined with different intervals between recording these signals (the time to echo or TE) yield images with various weighting and signal characteristics. Generally, when describing MRI sequences, we can refer to bright tissues or fluid as high intensity or dark tissues or fluid as low intensity. Typically, MRI scans are acquired at 1.5 or 3 Tesla (T). Increased field strength gives a higher signal-to-noise ratio but increases energy absorption and 3T scanners may not be suitable for patients with particular metallic implants or prosthesis. If there is any doubt, expert radiology advice is recommended.

MRI sequences

Soft-tissue contrast in MRI is related to differences in proton resonance within the tissues (fat and fluid). By changing MRI imaging parameters, differences in these properties can be emphasised; this is called weighting the image. Tissue can be characterised by two different relaxation times, T1 (longitudinal relaxation time) and T2 (transverse relaxation time). In general, T1- and T2-weighted images can be easily differentiated by looking at the cerebrospinal fluid (CSF). **CSF is dark on T1-weighted imaging (T1WI) and bright on T2-weighted imaging (T2WI)** (Figure 18.2).

T1-weighted image

• 'Short TR, short TE'
• Good for anatomical detail
• Water is dark, fat is bright

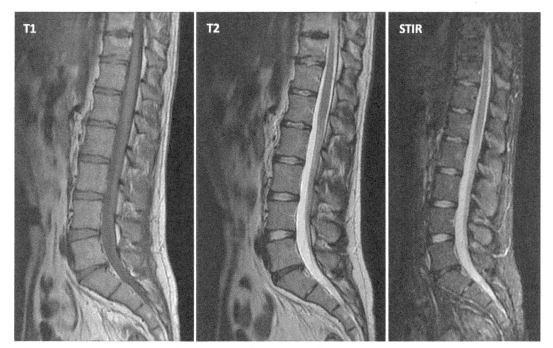

Figure 18.2 Sagittal spine MRI demonstrating the corresponding T1-weighted image, T2-weighted image and STIR image.

- Useful for assessing bone marrow, as any replacement of fatty marrow signal will appear dark (e.g. oedema, tumour infiltration, red marrow re-conversion)
- Poor detection of soft tissue oedema compared with T2WI

T2-weighted image

- 'Long TR, long TE'
- Detection of fluid and excellent detection of marrow pathology when combined with fat saturation
- Fluid and fat are bright
- Better for pathology, e.g. inflammation or oedema will appear high signal due to their fluid content

Proton density

- 'Intermediate TR, short TE'
- Weighted to reflect the density of protons and shares some features of both T1WI and T2WI

- Provides good anatomical detail but relatively little overall tissue contrast
  - Fluid (e.g. joint fluid, CSF): High signal intensity (white)
  - Muscle: Intermediate signal intensity (grey)
  - Fat: High signal intensity (white)

Fat suppression techniques

When fluid and fat are both bright, one option is to suppress the signal from fat, which accentuates the high signal coming from fluid, of which there are many different techniques. Short tau inversion recovery (STIR) is a fat-saturation technique that results in markedly decreased signal intensity from fat and increased signal from fluid and oedema making it a sensitive tool for identifying soft-tissue and marrow pathology (Figure 18.3).

- Bright T1 and T2 = Fat
- Bright T2 but dark STIR = Fat
- Bright T2 and bright STIR = Water/oedema

Figure 18.3 Simple schema to help differentiate fat and water/oedema from features on T1WI, T2WI and STIR sequences.

MUSCULOSKELETAL RADIOLOGY SPOT DIAGNOSES

SHOULDER AND UPPER LIMB

SHOULDER DISLOCATION

The humeral head is usually displaced medially with the humeral head and outline of the glenoid being incongruent (Figure 18.4). Ensure at least two views are obtained as some dislocations may not be obvious on one view only. Dislocations can also be identified on trans-scapular Y views. Assess for associated injuries, including Hill-Sachs lesion, Bankart lesion or proximal humeral fracture.

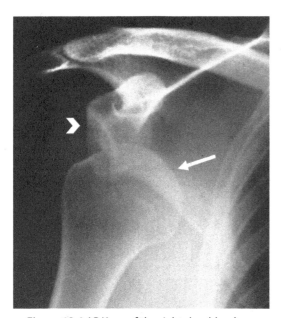

Figure 18.4 AP X-ray of the right shoulder demonstrating anterior shoulder dislocation. Note the medial displacement of the humeral head (*white arrow*) compared with the glenoid (*white arrowhead*). (Reproduced with kind permission from *Apley & Solomon's System of Orthopaedics and Trauma*, 10th edition, CRC Press, 2018.)

SUPERIOR LABRAL ANTERIOR POSTERIOR (SLAP) TEAR

MR arthrogram is the investigation of choice which demonstrates high signal (fluid on T2WI) extending and tracking into the superior labrum +/− biceps. Labrum is the dark triangle which is continuous with bone (Figure 18.5).

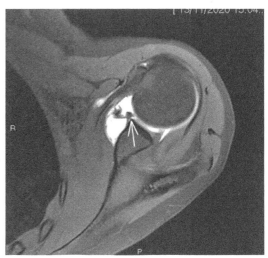

Figure 18.5 A 42 year old with a long history of left shoulder pain and instability. Axial MR arthrogram shows a SLAP lesion (*white arrow*) demonstrated by high signal extending and tracking into the superior labrum.

ROTATOR CUFF TEAR

Ultrasound (US) may show hypoechoic defects in the tendon, fluid along the biceps tendon or effusion in the subacromial/subdeltoid bursa or the glenohumeral joint. Indirect signs include a bright aspect of the humeral cartilage (cartilage interface sign). A full-thickness tear is a defect that reaches from the bursal to the articular margin. US is also useful to identify and potential differentials.

MRI may show a defect in the tendon filled with fluid in T2WI, tendon retraction +/− subdeltoid bursal effusion or fluid along the biceps (Figure 18.6). Muscle atrophy and fatty replacement is seen in chronic cases.

OSTEOCHONDRITIS DISSECANS OF THE CAPITELLAR JOINT

X-ray findings may be occult initially. Findings may include flattening or indistinct lucency around the contour surface (Figure 18.7). More advanced changes include fragmentation and density changes. MRI is the modality of choice with a high-intensity rim at the interface between the fragment and the bone on T2WI or a focal osteochondral defect filled with fluid if detached.

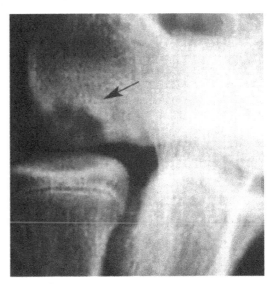

Figure 18.7 AP X-ray of the right elbow demonstrating contour abnormalities and low-density changes of the capitellum (*black arrow*). (Reproduced with kind permission from *Apley & Solomon's System of Orthopaedics and Trauma*, 10th edition, CRC Press, 2018.)

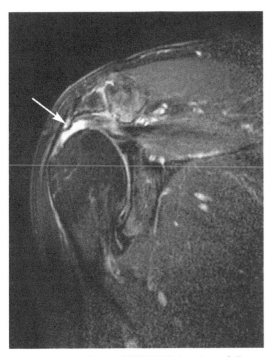

Figure 18.6 Coronal T2WI MRI showing a full-thickness tear of supraspinatus with tendon retraction. (Reproduced with kind permission from *Apley & Solomon's System of Orthopaedics and Trauma*, 10th edition, CRC Press, 2018.)

SCAPHOID FRACTURE

A standard set of X-rays should be taken for suspected scaphoid fracture consisting of four projections: posteroanterior (PA), oblique, lateral and posteroanterior view angled (known as Zitters – PA in ulnar deviation with 20° tube angulation of the elbow).

- PA view – best to inspect joint spaces of the carpal bones
- Oblique
- Lateral – fundamental view to assess for suspected dislocation
- PA angled – presents the scaphoid on its long axis (Figure 18.8)

Assess for fracture and displacement, displacement of adjacent fat pads and associated scapholunate ligament defect (Terry Thomas sign).

Plain radiographs may miss a significant number of acute scaphoid fractures. If no fracture is seen, but clinical suspicion is high, they should be immobilised and repeat radiographs performed in 7–10 days and/or MRI performed.

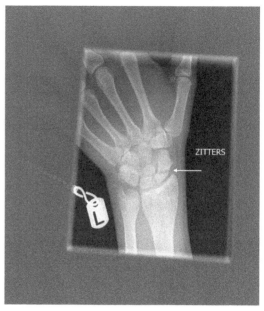

Figure 18.8 Zitters view radiograph of the scaphoid shows an undisplaced scaphoid waist fracture (*white arrow*).

SPINE

SPONDYLOLYSIS AND SPONDYLOLISTHESIS

X-rays are insensitive to early bone stress reactions. MRI has largely superseded other modalities and can also better evaluate disc degeneration and other causes of pain such as nerve root compression. Early stress reactions of the pars interarticularis can be visualised as bone marrow oedema on T2WI which appears as high intensity. The presence of a complete fracture is difficult to establish on routine MRI sequences and CT can be helpful to determine fracture lines (Figure 18.9). However, more recent 3T MRI with thin-slice T1WI volumetric interpolated breath-hold examination (VIBE) sequence has also shown to have comparable accuracy to CT in the detection and characterisation of incomplete pars stress fractures (1).

Spondylolisthesis is the slipping of one vertebra relative to the one below and is frequently a result of spondylolysis at L5/S1 or L4/L5. Lateral views on X-ray will show a forward shift of the upper part of the spinal column on the stable vertebra below (Figure 18.10). The degree of slip is measured by the amount of overlap of adjacent vertebral bodies and is expressed as a percentage (Meyerding classification).

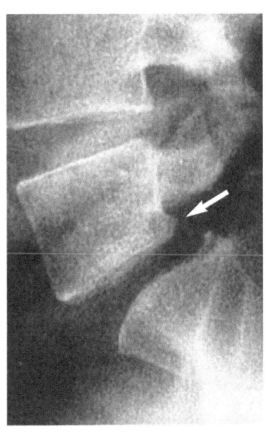

Figure 18.10 Lateral X-ray of the lumbar spine. There is a break in the pars interarticularis of L5 (*white arrow*), allowing the anterior part of the vertebra to slip forwards.

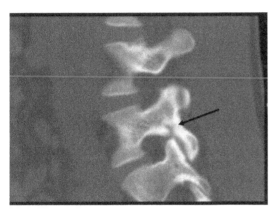

Figure 18.9 Sagittal CT of the lumbar spine in an elite footballer presenting with lower back pain, mid-season. Black arrow indicates the location of the stress lesion. (Reproduced with the kind permission of Professor Nick Peirce.)

ACUTE INTERVERTEBRAL DISC PROLAPSE

X-rays are helpful to exclude bony pathology. MRI is the default investigation of choice for spinal pathology. Disc herniation is the displacement of intervertebral disc material beyond the normal confines of the disc and can be divided into protrusions or extrusions. Sagittal T2WI images can give you the most diagnostic information. Once an abnormality is detected, correlate the findings with the T1WI images and the same level on the axial series (Figure 18.11).

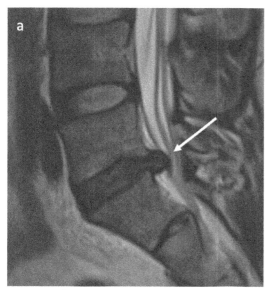

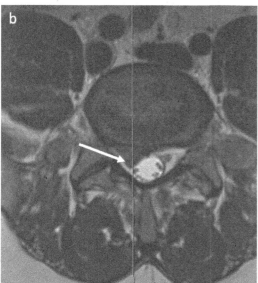

Figure 18.11 A T2WI MRI (a) sagittal and (b) axial views demonstrating L5/S1 right-sided disc protrusion (*white arrows*). (Reproduced with kind permission from *Apley & Solomon's System of Orthopaedics and Trauma*, 10th edition, CRC Press, 2018.)

CENTRAL CORD SYNDROME

X-ray and CT may show cervical spondylosis or an acute fracture. MRI will show increased signal in the cord at the level affected on T2 (Figure 18.12).

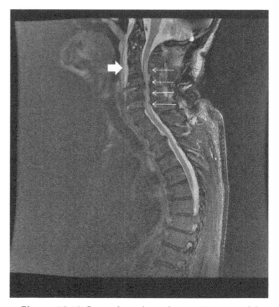

Figure 18.12 Central cord syndrome. 65-year-old patient with tetraplegia following a fall with a neck injury. Sagittal T2 fat-saturated (FS) MRI shows cord oedema extending from levels C2–C7 on a background of cervical canal stenosis (*arrows*). Prevertebral haematoma also noted at levels C2–C4 (*block arrow*).

HIP AND GROIN

FEMOROACETABULAR IMPINGEMENT (FAI)

In symptomatic patients, radiology can help to determine morphological variants of the femoral head/neck region and/or acetabulum. An AP X-ray of the pelvis and a cross-table lateral X-ray of the hip are first-line investigations. Abnormal signs related to acetabular over-coverage in pincer-type FAI include a crossover sign (Figure 18.13a). In cam-type FAI, there is a characteristic 'bump' at the superior head-neck junction that may be accompanied by a pistol-grip deformity of the proximal femur (Figure 18.13b). This can be assessed on a Dunn view by measuring the angle (alpha angle) between the orientation of the femoral neck and the margin of the femoral head. An alpha angle >50° would be abnormal.

AVULSION FRACTURE OF THE ANTERIOR SUPERIOR ILIAC SPINE

Acute avulsion injuries can be identified on X-rays as avulsed bone fragments. Sudden eccentric contraction and forceful extension of the hip, e.g. in sprinters, can cause a common avulsion at the anterior superior iliac spine (ASIS), which is the site of the attachment of sartorius and the tensor fascia lata (Figure 18.14). Distinct margins of the fracture help to determine the acute nature of these injuries compared with chronic ones.

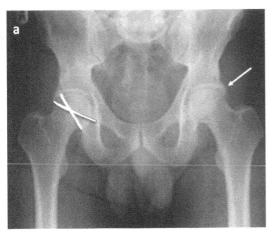

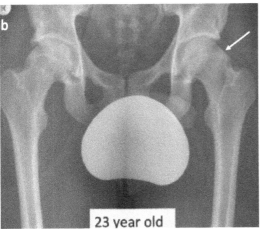

Figure 18.13 (a) AP X-ray of the pelvis showing a positive crossover sign (depicted with white lines on the right side) in pincer-type FAI indicating acetabular retroversion. A line drawn down the anterior wall will intersect with a line drawn along the posterior wall. Focal anterior acetabular over-coverage indicated with white arrow on the left. (b) AP X-ray of the pelvis showing predominantly cam-type FAI indicated by a loss of sphericity of the femoral head and characteristic cam lesion or 'bump' at the superior head-neck junction (*white arrow*).

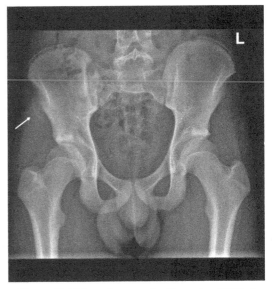

Figure 18.14 Anterior superior iliac spine (ASIS). A 14 year old who presented after feeling a sudden 'snap' over their right hip on running. AP X-ray of the pelvis shows an acute avulsion fracture of the right ASIS (*white arrow*). There are bilateral unfused iliac crest apophyses due to the age of the patient.

FEMORAL NECK STRESS FRACTURE

X-rays can detect established stress fractures (>6 weeks), but MRI is the best modality to identify associated bone marrow oedema and early changes. MRI would show a linear hypointense fracture line with associated surrounding marrow oedema +/− soft tissue oedema (Figure 18.15). Note if the location is inferior (low risk) or superior (high risk).

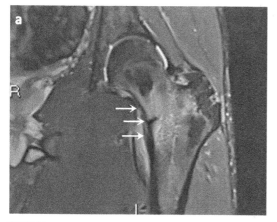

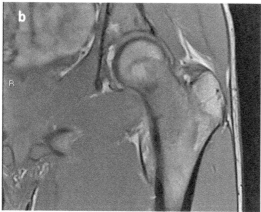

Figure 18.15 A 22-year-old triathlete presenting with left hip pain. (a) Coronal STIR shows a left femoral neck stress fracture (*middle arrow*) with surrounding oedema (*adjacent arrows*). (b) Appearances of the stress fracture on corresponding T1WI.

SLIPPED UPPER FEMORAL EPIPHYSIS (SUFE)

Plain X-rays are the key diagnostic imaging tool in children with suspected SUFE. Initial views should include AP and frog-lateral of both hips (Figure 18.16a). Lateral views are more sensitive for early signs of a slip, including widening of the physis, loss of the anterior head-neck concavity and loss of total epiphyseal height. MRI is useful where there is high clinical suspicion with negative radiographs. There are several ways to objectively measure physeal slip. Klein's line is a line drawn on the AP radiograph along the superior border of the neck. If this line fails to intersect the epiphysis or intersects a smaller portion of the epiphysis compared with this other side, this is a positive Trethowan sign and may indicate a slip (Figure 18.16b).

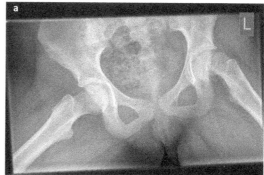

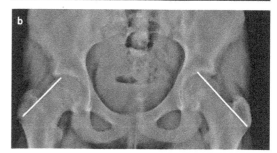

Figure 18.16 (a) A 12 year old with left-sided hip pain. Frog leg lateral view shows a left-sided slipped upper femoral epiphysis. (b) AP radiograph of a different patient, with Klein's lines drawn bilaterally with a positive Trethowan sign in the right hip.

HAMSTRING TEAR

MRI is the investigation of choice to determine the size and location of the muscle tear. On T2-weighted images, the principal finding is hyperintensity of the injured area suggestive of oedema, most commonly of the musculotendinous junction (MTJ) (Figure 18.17). Architectural disruption and tendon involvement is often commented on, as well as the absence or presence of haematoma formation. MRI is superior to US in identifying deep structures and determining acute from chronic tears.

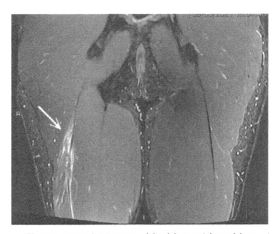

Figure 18.17 A 20-year-old athlete with sudden onset hamstring pain whilst training. Coronal STIR of the hamstring shows an acute tear of the right biceps femoris with tendon involvement (*white arrow*). A normal left biceps femoris is also imaged for comparison.

KNEE

ANTERIOR CRUCIATE LIGAMENT TEAR

X-rays may demonstrate secondary features such as a Segond fracture (avulsion of lateral collateral band), joint effusion or anterior tibial translation.

MRI is the imaging modality of choice.

On sagittal view, look for:

- A tendon that does not align with the inter-condylar (Blumensaat's) line
- Discontinuity of fibres on T2WI (Figure 18.18a)

- A wavy tendon
- Associated bone oedema

On coronal T2-weighted image, i.e. proton density fat saturated (PDFS) or STIR, look for:

- 'Empty notch sign' which is typical for proximal tear and indicates fluid against the lateral wall (Figure 18.18b)

Other secondary signs include anterior tibial translation and bone oedema which can persist for 6 weeks in the lateral femoral condyle and posterior tibial plateau. Assess closely for associated injuries such as to the menisci or collateral ligaments.

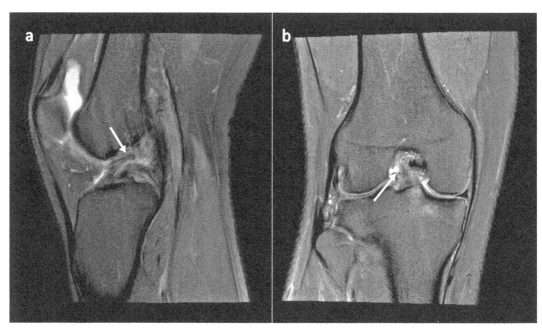

Figure 18.18 A 33 year old with a history of twisting their knee. (a) Sagittal PDFS shows a complete ACL rupture (*white arrow*) demonstrated by discontinuity of the fibres. (b) Appearances of the ACL rupture on coronal PDFS demonstrating fluid against the lateral wall or an 'empty notch sign'.

BUCKET HANDLE MENISCAL TEAR

Acute meniscal tears of the knee are best evaluated using MRI. Bucket handle tears are full-thickness displaced vertical meniscal tears, in which there is central displacement of the inner part, but the separated fragment remains attached front and back. Radiological signs include:

- A double PCL sign on sagittal view (medial meniscus; Figure 18.19a)
- A double ACL sign on sagittal view (lateral meniscus)
- Absent bow tie sign on sagittal view
- Meniscal fragment in the intercondylar notch on coronal view (Figure 18.19b)

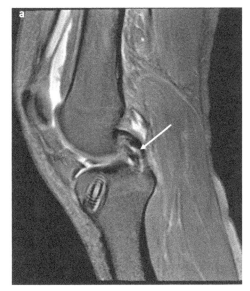

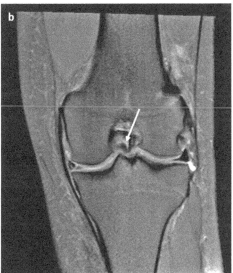

Figure 18.19 A 27 year old with previous ACL reconstruction, presents with a history of twisting their knee with persistent pain and locking. (a) Sagittal PDFS shows a 'double PCL sign' consistent with a bucket handle tear of the medial meniscus (*white arrow*). (b) Coronal PDFS shows the displaced meniscal fragment at the intercondylar notch (*white arrow*).

PATELLAR DISLOCATION

On axial MRI views, look for a 'kissing contusion pattern' indicating bone marrow oedema on medial patella and lateral femoral condyle (Figure 18.20). Check to see if the medial patellofemoral ligament (MPFL) is intact.

You can assess for risk factors for dislocation which may assist in guiding management.

Check bony anatomy on X-ray using AP, lateral and sunrise views.

- Lateral: Trochlear dysplasia (crossing sign or double contour sign) and patellar height (Insall-Salvati 0.8–1.2)
- Sunrise: Shallow trochlear groove <3 mm, small medial trochlear facet and lateral patellar tilt (lateral patellofemoral [PF] angle normally >11°)

On CT or MRI axial images:

- Lateralisation of the tibial tuberosity (TT): Tibial tuberosity to trochlear groove (TT-TG) distance (>20 mm abnormal)

On lateral X-ray or sagittal MRI:

- Patella alta – check for patella tendon length: Patella height or Insall-Salvati ratio >1.2 indicates patella alta; Figure 18.21)

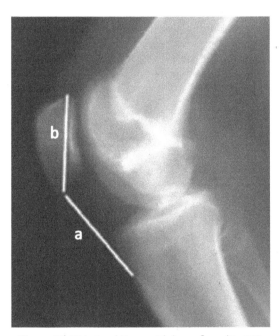

Figure 18.21 Lateral X-ray with knee flexed to 30°. (a) The length of the patellar tendon which is the length of the posterior surface of the tendon from the lower pole of the patella to its insertion on the tibia and (b) the patellar length which is the greatest pole-to-pole length. The Insall-Salvati ratio is calculated as a/b.

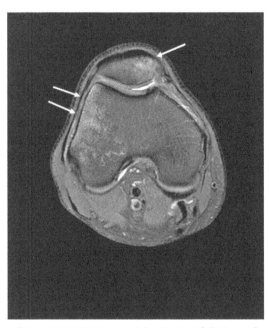

Figure 18.20 A 22-year-old patient with history of recent patellar dislocation. Axial PDFS showing marrow oedema within the medial patellar facet (single *white arrow*) and the lateral femoral condyle (double *white arrows*).

OSTEOCHONDRAL DEFECT OF THE KNEE

MRI is the optimum modality to assess changes and degree of fragment separation which will guide future management. Displaced lesions can be detected by high signal between fragment and adjacent bone on T2WI, the presence of high signal subchondral cysts beneath the lesion, or a focal osteochondral defect (Figure 18.22a).

X-ray: (AP, lateral and notch view) may miss early changes. Assess for subtle flattening or indistinct radiolucency around the cortical surface (Figure 18.22b) or Frank fragmentation.

OSTEOARTHRITIS OF THE KNEE

Pathognomonic features on X-ray are joint space narrowing, osteophyte formation, subchondral sclerosis and bone cysts. The medial compartment is more commonly affected than the lateral compartment (Figure 18.23).

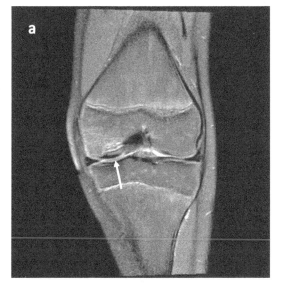

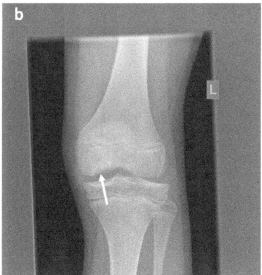

Figure 18.22 A 15 year old presenting with several months of left knee pain. (a) Coronal PDFS shows a detached but undisplaced osteochondral fragment with surrounding oedema (*white arrow*). This corresponds with a type III osteochondral injury as per the Clanton classification. (b) AP radiograph showing the same osteochondral fragment characterised by flattening and radiolucency at the cortical surface (*white arrow*).

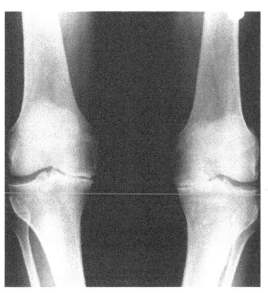

Figure 18.23 AP X-ray of the knees revealing bilateral reduction of the medial joint space and subchondral sclerosis. (Reproduced with kind permission from *Apley & Solomon's System of Orthopaedics and Trauma*, 10th edition, CRC Press, 2018.)

MYOSITIS OSSIFICANS

X-rays will demonstrate fluffy density in the soft tissue adjacent to the bone (Figure 18.24a). Other features include circumferential calcification with a lucent centre. CT can also demonstrate mineralisation (Figure 18.24b) and MRI may be helpful to differentiate from malignancy. Differentials would include osteosarcoma or soft tissue sarcoma.

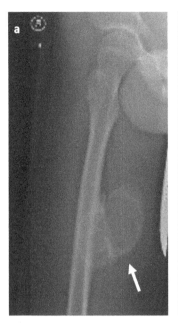 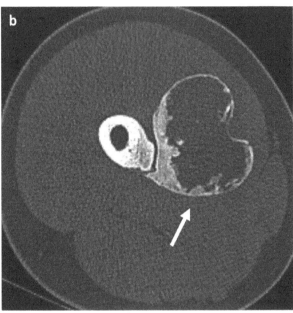

Figure 18.24 A 13-year-old boy presented with a painful mass in the adductor compartment of the right thigh after receiving a dead leg playing rugby a few months earlier. (a) An X-ray of the right femur demonstrating a large opacification within the medial thigh but separate from the femur with periosteal calcification (*white arrow*). (b) Axial CT in the same patient which confirms the calcific mass (*white arrow*) with a clear plane between the lesion and the femur. (Reproduced with kind permission from *Apley & Solomon's System of Orthopaedics and Trauma*, 10th edition, CRC Press, 2018.)

FOOT AND ANKLE

LATERAL LIGAMENT COMPLEX INJURIES

The anterior tibiofibular ligament (ATFL) is the most commonly injured ligament of the lateral ankle ligament complex. US or MRI has high sensitivity and specificity. MRI may show discontinuity of the ligament, detachment, contour irregularity or intrasubstance oedema (Figure 18.25).

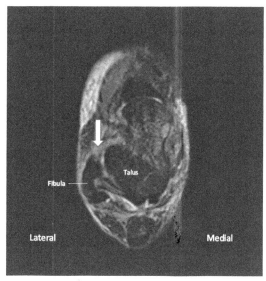

Figure 18.25 A 37-year-old male presenting with instability following an inversion injury. Axial STIR shows a full-thickness tear of the ATFL (*white arrow*).

MIDPORTION ACHILLES TENDINOPATHY

Ultrasound may show thickening of the tendon, hypoechoic portions and neovascularisation (Figure 18.26). MRI will demonstrate high signal, tendon enlargement and possibly partial tears (Figure 18.27).

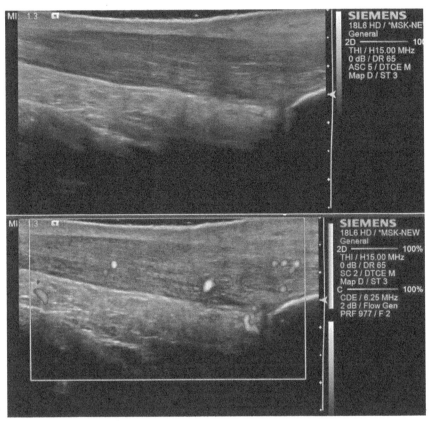

Figure 18.26 A 45-year-old patient presenting with a painful Achilles. Longitudinal ultrasound shows thickening and heterogenous echotexture of the tendon (*top image*) with neovascularity demonstrated on Doppler (*bottom image*).

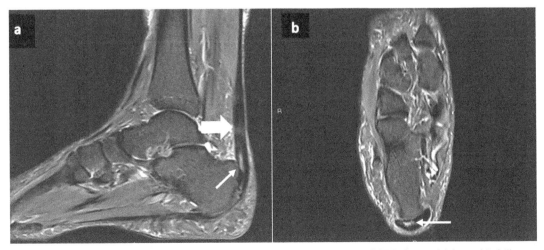

Figure 18.27 A 32-year-old patient with chronic Achilles pain. (a) Sagittal STIR shows thickened Achilles tendon (*thick white arrow*) with a partial thickness intrasubstance tear (*smaller white arrow*). (b) Axial STIR demonstrating the intrasubstance tear (*white arrow*).

ANTERIOR ANKLE IMPINGEMENT

Anterior ankle impingement is common in sports where there is repetitive dorsiflexion. Lateral ankle X-rays will show bony exostoses at the anterior tibial margin (Figure 18.28).

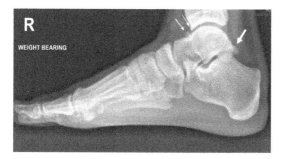

Figure 18.28 Footballer with anterior ankle joint pain and limited dorsiflexion. Lateral X-ray shows osteophytic tibiotalar spurs as a result of chronic repetitive trauma (double white arrows). Note, there is also an asymptomatic Os Trigonum (single thick *white arrow*).

TARSAL COALITION

X-rays are first line and should include AP, standing lateral, Harris views (axial calcaneal projection) and 45° internal oblique view.

- Calcaneonavicular coalition may be demonstrated with an 'anteater sign' (Figure 18.29) which refers to an anterior elongation of the superior calcaneus which overlaps the navicular on lateral X-ray
- Talocalcaneal coalition may be demonstrated on lateral X-ray with a talar beak or characteristic 'c-sign' which is an arc formed by the medial outline of the talar dome and posteroinferior aspect of sustentaculum tali

CT can help to determine the size and location of the coalition whilst MRI is useful to visualise cartilaginous or fibrous bridges.

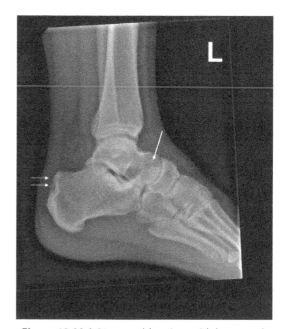

Figure 18.29 A 31-year-old patient with longstanding midfoot and Achilles insertional pain. Lateral radiograph shows the 'anteater sign' of calcaneonavicular coalition (single *white arrow*). There is also enthesitis at the site of the insertion of the Achilles (double *white arrows*).

RED FLAG PATHOLOGY NOT TO MISS

SPONDYLOARTHROPATHY

MRI of the sacroiliac joints (SIJ) and whole spine is now the gold standard for identifying changes consistent with Spondyloarthropathy, in particular, early lesions prior to new bone formation. Specialist sequencing protocols such as fat-suppressed T2WI or high-resolution STIR will show active inflammation suggestive of sacroiliitis +/− corner lesions (Figure 18.30a and b). Chronic changes include fatty replacement (high T1WI and T2WI) and sclerosis (low signal T1WI and T2WI).

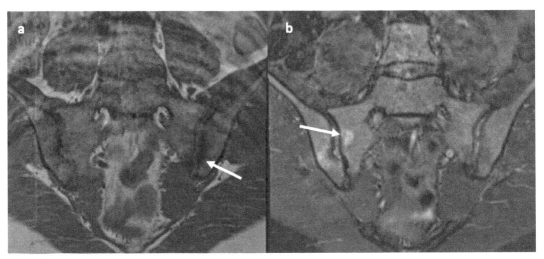

Figure 18.30 (a) Midcoronal oblique T1-weighted image of the SIJ demonstrating articular surface irregularity, subchondral sclerosis, joint space widening on the left, tissue backfill on the right. (b) Midcoronal oblique STIR image of SIJ demonstrating subchondral bone marrow oedema involving both the sacral and iliac joint surfaces. Focal erosion is noted involving the iliac articular surface with articular irregularity and surrounding bone marrow oedema. Tissue backfill with increased T2WI signal intensity is noted more marked on the right.

OSTEOMYELITIS

X-rays may have subtle early changes including loss or blurring of normal fat planes. After approximately 7 days, changes may include a periosteal reaction, focal bony lysis and endosteal scalloping (Figures 18.31a and b). MRI is the most sensitive and can delineate soft tissue expansion (Figure 18.31c). Bone marrow oedema can be detected on MRI after only 1 to 2 days of infection. Use of gadolinium contrast can also be helpful when infection is suspected. Suspected cases will require orthopaedic referral for aspiration of fluid from the metaphyseal subperiosteal abscess, extraosseous soft tissues or an adjacent joint and analysed for cell differential, organisms and sensitivity to antibiotics.

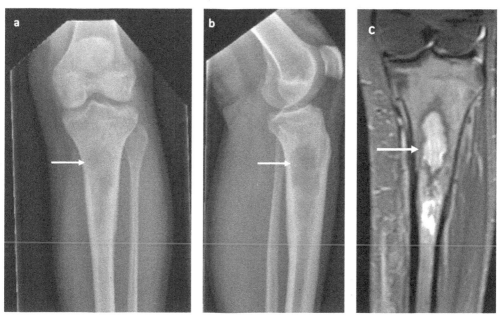

Figure 18.31 A 29 year old presented with rapidly progressive pain in the proximal tibia with general malaise and fever. Blood tests showed a raised C-reactive protein (CRP) and erythrocyte sedimentation rate (ESR). (a) AP and (b) lateral X-ray demonstrate a lytic expansile lesion in the proximal tibia (*white arrow*). (c) Coronal MRI demonstrates a fluid-filled cavity in the proximal tibial metaphysis with rim enhancement and florid perilesional oedema (*white arrow*) but without expansion into the periosteum or soft tissues. (Reproduced with kind permission from *Apley & Solomon's System of Orthopaedics and Trauma*, 10th edition, CRC Press, 2018.)

MALIGNANCY

OSTEOSARCOMA

Osteosarcoma is the most common primary malignant bone tumour. The majority present at the distal femur, proximal tibia or humerus and pathological fracture is rare. X-rays are generally diagnostic demonstrating ill-defined, permeative bone-forming lesions with cortical destruction, periosteal reaction and soft-tissue expansion.

Rapidly enlarging subperiosteal lesions may elevate the periosteum so quickly that bone deposition occurs only at the margins, creating a Codman's triangle (Figure 18.32a). Attempts at bone formation may produce streaks of calcification termed sunray spicules. These findings can also be seen with Ewing sarcoma, chondrosarcoma, metastasis and malignant giant cell tumour. MRI can delineate the full extent of the tumour and extension into surrounding soft tissues (Figure 18.32b).

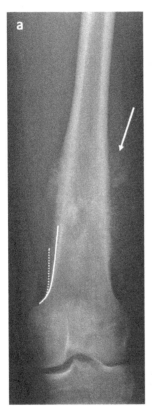 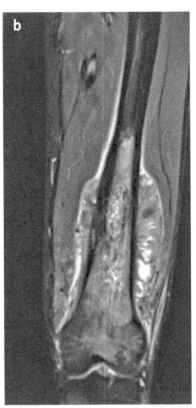

Figure 18.32 (a) AP X-ray of the distal femur showing an osteosarcoma in the metadiaphysis which demonstrates a mixed lytic blastic appearance with elevation of the periosteum resulting in a Codman's triangle (dotted white line). The soft-tissue extension of the tumour results in new bone formation within the surrounding tissues and appearances of sunray spiculations (*white arrow*). (b) Coronal T2FS MRI demonstrates the true extent of the lesion with tumour erupting from the bone and extending into the surrounding soft tissues. (Reproduced with kind permission from *Apley & Solomon's System of Orthopaedics and Trauma*, 10th edition, CRC Press, 2018.)

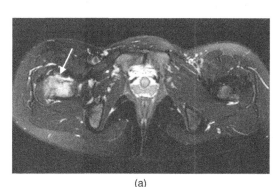

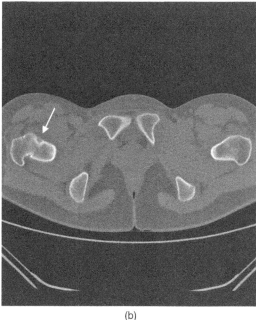

(a)   (b)

Figure 18.33 A 17 year old with a several month history of right hip pain. (a) Axial PDFS shows non-specific marrow oedema within the right neck of femur (*white arrow*). (b) Axial CT shows an anterior cortical-based lucent lesion surrounded by a rim of sclerosis (*white arrow*) consistent with an osteoid osteoma.

OSTEOID OSTEOMA

These are small, benign tumours formed of osteoid and woven bone surrounded by a halo of reactive bone. They are common in young patients and in long bones. X-rays demonstrate an area of dense sclerosis with a small, rounded area of osteolysis which may be obscured by surrounding sclerosis. MRI is sensitive but non-specific for osteoid osteoma (Figure 18.33a). The central nidus of the lesion is best seen on CT scan (Figure 18.33b). Preferred treatment is CT-guided radiofrequency ablation.

REFERENCE

1. Ang EC, Robertson AF, Malara FA, O'Shea T, Roebert JK, Schneider ME, et al. Diagnostic accuracy of 3-T magnetic resonance imaging with 3D T1 VIBE versus computer tomography in pars stress fracture of the lumbar spine. *Skeletal Radiol.* 2016;45:1533–40.

Index

Note: Locators in *italics* represent figures and **bold** indicate tables in the text.